Paediatric Immediate Life Support

4th Edition, May 2021

Reprinted March 2022

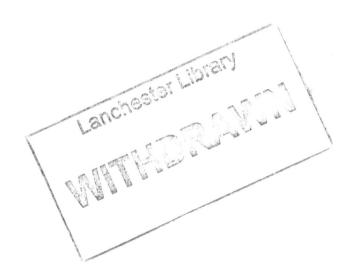
PILS

Paediatric Immediate Life Support
4th Edition, May 2021
Reprinted March 2022

ISBN 978-1-903812-38-9

Published by © Resuscitation Council UK 2021
5th Floor, Tavistock House North, Tavistock Square, London WC1H 9HR
Tel: 020 7388 4678 email: enquiries@resus.org.uk www.resus.org.uk

Printed by All About Print.
Tel: 020 7205 4022 email: hello@allaboutprint.co.uk www.allaboutprint.co.uk
Printed on responsibly sourced environmentally friendly paper made with elemental chlorine free fibre from legal and sustainably managed forests.

Photographs © Resuscitation Council UK

Photography by Ed Tyler, Mark Sedge and Ashley Prytherch
Colour plates reproduced with permission of the Northern Neonatal Network who retain copyright.

Electrical conduction of the heart (Figure 7.2) © LifeART image (1989–2001) Wolters Kluwer Health, Inc.-Lippincott Williams & Wilkins. All rights reserved.

Design and artwork by Fruition London
www.fruitionlondon.com

The Resuscitation Council UK guidelines are adapted from the European Resuscitation Council guidelines and have been developed using a process accredited by The National Institute for Health and Care Excellence. The UK guidelines are consistent with the European guidelines but include minor modifications to reflect the needs of the National Health Service.

This Paediatric Immediate Life Support (PILS) manual is written by the Resuscitation Council UK EPALS Subcommittee and forms part of the resources for the Resuscitation Council UK PILS course, which is delivered in accredited course centres throughout the UK.

Acknowledgements

We thank and acknowledge the members of the ERC 2021 Guidelines Writing Group who have contributed directly or indirectly to this PILS Manual.

We thank the Nuffield Hospital, Guildford, for the use of their facilities, the Royal Surrey NHS Foundation Trust, specifically the Resuscitation Department for their assistance with photography, Lifecast Body Simulation for the loan of manikins and all the Instructors who gave up their time to take part in the photography shoot.

We thank Oliver Meyer for digital preparation of the rhythm strips,

We thank Ed Tyler, Ashley Prytherch and Mark Sedge for the photography taken and digitally prepared for the manual.

Previous contributors

Ben Lakin
Sarah Mitchell
Liz Norris
Ruchi Sinha
Felicity Todd
Mark Woolcock
Jonathan Wyllie

Authors

Liesje Andre
Marion De Almeida Santos
Adam Benson Clarke
Robert Bingham
Mandy Brailsford
Fiona Clements
Mike Coren
Jane Davies
Isabelle Hamilton-Bower
Sue Hampshire
Mae Johnson
Ralph Mackinnon
Ian Maconochie
Ian McDougall
Sophie Skellett
Denise Welsby
Mark Worrall
Deborah Zeitlin

Editors

Sophie Skellett
Liesje Andre
Adam Benson Clarke
Fiona Clements
Isabelle Hamilton-Bower
Sue Hampshire
Ian McDougall

Contents

Contents

Notes

Glossary

Abbreviation	In full
AED	automated external defibrillator
BLS	basic life support
BMV	bag-mask ventilation
BP	blood pressure
CO	cardiac output
CO_2	carbon dioxide
CPR	cardiopulmonary resuscitation
CRT	capillary refill time
ECG	electrocardiogram
EPALS	european paediatric advanced life support
EMS	emergency medical service (e.g. ambulance service)
$ETCO_2$	end-tidal carbon dioxide
FEV	forced expiratory volume
FiO_2	fraction of inspired oxygen
HR	heart rate
h	hours
IM	intramuscular
IO	intraosseous
IV	intravenous
O_2	oxygen
$PaCO_2$	partial pressure of arterial carbon dioxide
min	minutes
PEA	pulseless electrical activity
PEEP	positive end expiratory pressure
PEF	peak expiratory flow
PICU	paediatric intensive care unit
ROSC	return of spontaneous circulation
RR	respiratory rate
SaO_2	arterial oxygen saturation
s	seconds
SpO_2	peripheral arterial oxygen saturation from an oximeter probe
SV	stroke volume
SVR	systemic vascular resistance
SVT	supraventricular tachycardia
Tidal volume	volume of each breath
TT	tracheal tube
VF	ventricular fibrillation
pVT	pulseless VT
VT	ventricular tachycardia
<	less than
≤	less than or equal to
>	greater than
≥	greater than or equal to

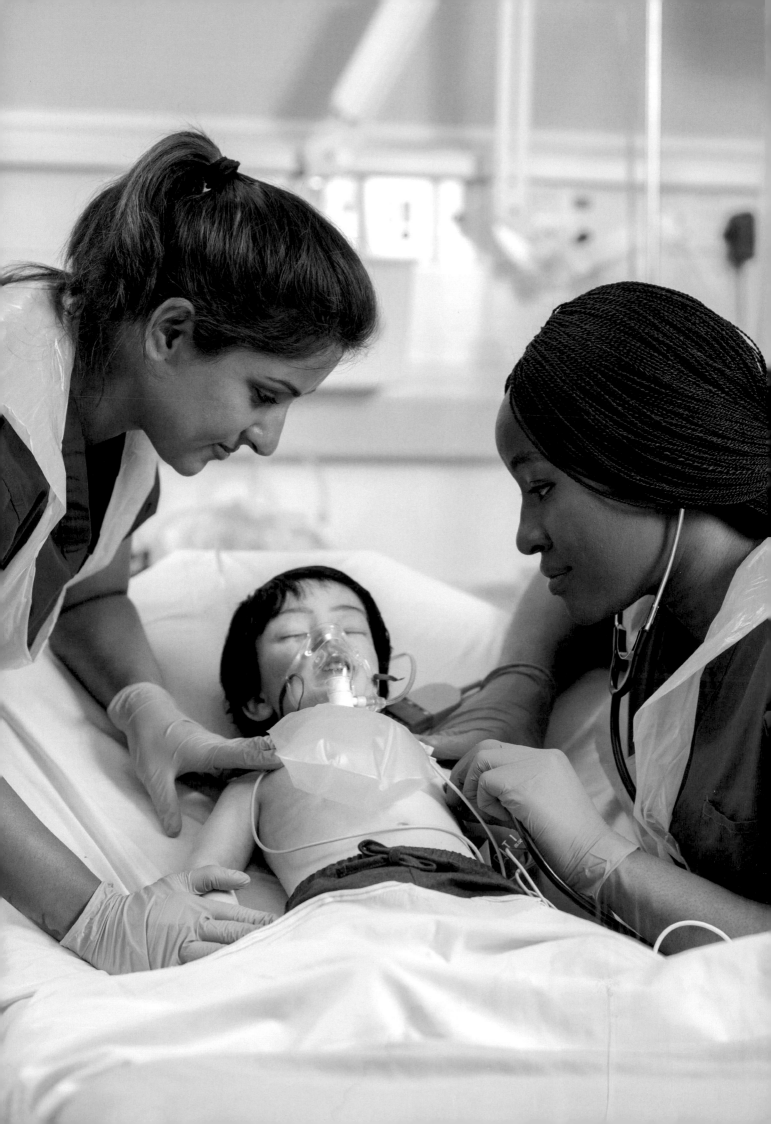

Introduction to Paediatric Immediate Life Support

01

Aetiologies of cardiorespiratory arrest

The aetiology of cardiorespiratory arrest in children differs from adults. This is due to anatomical, physiological and pathological differences, which alter throughout childhood.

Primary cardiorespiratory arrest is a sudden acute event, which occurs without warning. It is commonly due to a cardiac arrhythmia reflecting intrinsic heart disease. A successful outcome is generally dependent on rapid defibrillation, as the most common arrhythmias encountered in primary cardiorespiratory arrests are ventricular fibrillation (VF) or pulseless ventricular tachycardia (pVT). Every minute of delay until defibrillation results in the number of successful cases with a return of spontaneous circulation (ROSC) decreasing by approximately 10%.

A primary cardiac arrest is most common in adults but can occur in older children or children with congenital heart disease. Overall, however, the most common cause of cardiorespiratory arrest in children is secondary to other intercurrent illnesses.

Secondary cardiorespiratory arrest is usually due to hypoxia and reflects the limit of the body's ability to compensate for the effects of underlying illness or injury. Severe tissue hypoxia causes myocardial dysfunction, resulting in profound bradycardia, which typically deteriorates to asystole or pulseless electrical activity (PEA). Both PEA and asystole are associated with a poor outcome.

Secondary cardiorespiratory arrest is rarely a sudden event but follows a progressive deterioration. As respiratory and circulatory failure worsen (Figure 1.1), the body initially activates adaptive physiological responses compensating for the effects of the deterioration on vital organs (compensated respiratory or circulatory failure). These adaptive responses result in signs and symptoms that can be recognised, thereby providing an opportunity to intervene before further deterioration to cardiorespiratory arrest.

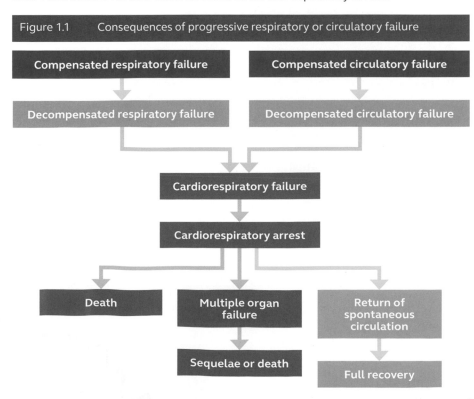

Figure 1.1   Consequences of progressive respiratory or circulatory failure

Outcome from secondary cardiorespiratory arrest

The outcome from secondary cardiorespiratory arrest is poor. Severe tissue hypoxia occurring before the heart stops means that all the vital organs are potentially seriously compromised; the heart finally arrests as a result of severe myocardial hypoxia.

Even if ROSC is achieved, morbidity and mortality remains high. Rates of successful resuscitation from out-of-hospital cardiorespiratory arrest (OHCA) are low (4–12% survival), and less than 5% of children will survive without neurological sequelae. In-hospital cardiorespiratory arrest (IHCA) results are better with a 60–80% ROSC rate, but many children succumb to severe organ injury (e.g. brain, kidney) or multi-system organ failure 48–72 h post-arrest. Data from the National Cardiac Arrest Audit (NCAA) in the UK between 2012–2018 indicated that 69% of patients achieved ROSC, but only 54% of children survived to hospital discharge following IHCA in this time period.

Resuscitation from respiratory arrest, when there is still cardiac output, is associated with much better (80–90%) good quality, long-term survival.

Anatomical and physiological considerations

The underlying anatomical and physiological differences between infants, young children and adults largely account for the difference in aetiology of cardiorespiratory arrest.

The key differences will be considered in order of management priority based on the ABCDE approach.

A	Airway
B	Breathing
C	Circulation
D	Disability (mental status)
E	Exposure

A Airway

The infant/young child has an airway that is proportionately narrower and more susceptible to oedema and swelling than the adult. The absolute diameter of the airway is also smaller, and therefore respiratory infections account for a significantly higher level of morbidity and mortality in young children.

Relationship between head and neck

The infant's head is large in relation to the rest of their body. Since the occiput is protuberant, the head tends to flex on the neck when the infant is placed in a supine position. This leads to potential obstruction of the airway when the conscious level is reduced. With increasing age, the child's head becomes smaller in relation to their thorax, the neck lengthens, and the larynx becomes more resistant to external pressure as tissues become less compliant. This explains why airway opening positions are different at different ages.

Face and mouth

The infant's face is small, and therefore the sizing of a face mask needs to be accurate; otherwise, it is difficult to achieve an effective seal. Additionally, pressure to the eyes can lead to damage and reflex bradycardia and must be avoided.

Inside the small mouth, the tongue is relatively large. This combination means that airway obstruction is more likely in the unconscious infant/young child. The floor of the mouth is easily compressible; care is required to avoid compressing the soft tissues under the mandible to prevent airway obstruction when performing airway manoeuvres.

Nose and pharynx

The infant is a preferential nasal breather for the first six months or so of life. As a result, anything that causes nasal obstruction (e.g. anatomical abnormalities such as choanal atresia, copious secretions, nasogastric tubes or tapes) can lead to increased work of breathing and respiratory compromise.

The epiglottis in infants is larger and floppier than in adults. This means that it is vulnerable to damage by airway devices and manoeuvres; additionally, manipulation of the epiglottis can lead to vagal stimulation.

The larynx

The larynx is higher in the infant compared to the older child and adult (where it is level with C5–6). The anatomical variations have the following practical implications:

- Blind finger sweeps to remove a foreign body must not be performed in young children with partial airway obstruction as these may convert a partial into a complete obstruction. The foreign body can become impacted into the narrowest part of the larynx.

- The relatively large tongue may create airway obstruction as the epiglottis and larynx are higher in the neck.

- Control of the large tongue with a laryngoscope blade may be difficult.

- The high position of the larynx in an infant creates a sharp angle between the oropharynx and the glottis. Direct visualisation of the glottis with the laryngoscope is therefore difficult. It may be easier to use a straight blade rather than a curved blade to obtain a view, particularly in infants up to three months of age (this does, however, result in more vagal stimulation).

B Breathing

Physiological considerations

Infants and small children have a relatively small resting lung volume and hence a low oxygen reserve. In addition, they have a high rate of oxygen consumption. This combination results in rapid falls in blood oxygen levels when respiration is compromised.

Spontaneous tidal volume stays constant throughout life at 4–6 mL kg^{-1}. It can be qualitatively assessed by auscultation of the chest, listening to air entry in the upper and lower zones of both sides of the chest.

Mechanics of breathing

As they age, the mechanics of children's breathing changes. The infant has ribs that are cartilaginous and pliable, while their intercostal muscles are weak and relatively ineffective. The main muscle of respiration is the diaphragm. During inspiration, the diaphragm descends towards the abdomen, generating a negative pressure, which draws air into the upper airway and the lungs.

Mechanical impedance to the contraction of the diaphragm (e.g. gastric distension, intestinal obstruction) will result in ineffective ventilation, as will any obstruction of the airway (e.g. bronchiolitis, asthma or foreign body aspiration).

In older children, the more developed intercostal muscles contribute significantly to the mechanics of breathing. The ribs ossify and act as a secure anchor for the muscles, as well as forming a more rigid structure that is less likely to collapse in respiratory distress. In children above five years, the presence of significant intercostal recession should therefore be considered as an ominous sign and indicative of serious respiratory compromise.

Respiratory rate

Normal respiration requires minimal effort, and the resting respiratory rate varies with age. The infant has a relatively high metabolic rate, O_2 consumption and CO_2 production, which is the main reason for their increased respiratory rates (Table 1.1). The respiratory rate also increases with agitation, anxiety and the presence of fever; therefore, a record of respiratory rate as it changes over time is more useful than a single value.

Table 1.1 Respiratory rate ranges by age

Age (years)	Respiratory rate (breaths min^{-1})
< 1	30–40 min^{-1}
1–2	26–34 min^{-1}
2–5	24–30 min^{-1}
5–12	20–24 min^{-1}
> 12	12–20 min^{-1}

C Circulation

The circulating volume of the newborn is 80 mL kg^{-1} and decreases with age to 60–70 mL kg^{-1} in adulthood. This means that the total circulating volume of an infant is very small (e.g. 240 mL in a newborn of 3 kg and 480 mL in a six-month-old with a weight of 6 kg). Relatively small losses can be a significantly high percentage of their total circulating volume; this is why apparently minor diarrhoeal illnesses can result in considerable morbidity and even mortality in infants and young children.

Heart rate

Stroke volume (i.e. the amount of blood ejected with each contraction of the heart) is relatively small in infancy, (1.5 mL kg^{-1} at birth) and increases along with heart size. However, the cardiac output relative to body weight is higher than at any other stage of life (300 mL kg^{-1} min^{-1}, decreasing to 100 mL kg^{-1} min^{-1} in adolescence and 70–80 mL kg^{-1} min^{-1} in adults).

Cardiac output

Cardiac output is the product of stroke volume and heart rate, and so the high cardiac outputs in infants and young children are primarily achieved by rapid heart rates (Table 1.2).

$$CO = HR \times SV$$

CO = Cardiac output

HR = Heart Rate

SV = Stroke Volume (blood volume ejected with each contraction)

Table 1.2   Heart rate ranges (beats min^{-1})

Age	Mean	Awake	Deep sleep
Newborn – 3 months	140	85–205	80–140
3 months – 2 years	130	100–180	75–160
2–10 years	80	60–140	60–90
> 10 years	75	60–100	50–90

Since cardiac output is directly related to the heart rate, bradycardia is a serious event and should be treated vigorously.

Systemic vascular resistance increases as the child ages, and this is reflected in the changes seen in blood pressure (BP) ranges (Table 1.3).

In sick children and infants, it is useful to consider the mean arterial blood pressure as an indicator of blood flow, and it is believed to be a better indicator of tissue perfusion than systolic BP (as it accounts for the fact that two-thirds of the cardiac cycle is spent in diastole).

Mean arterial pressure (MAP) is derived from a patient's systolic blood pressure (SBP) and diastolic blood pressure (DBP). Since MAP is a product of cardiac output (CO) and systemic vascular resistance (SVR) (MAP = CO x SVR), variations in SVR make the relationship between MAP and CO often unreliable (e.g. a patient with a poor CO but high SVR such as a patient in cardiogenic shock may have an acceptable MAP but a CO that is too low to provide adequate perfusion to tissues). The MAP should be calculated in acute conditions by the method below and compared to the MAP expected (Table 1.3).

$$((2 \times \text{diastolic}) + \text{systolic}) / 3 = \text{MAP (mmHg)}$$

D Disability

The limited communication skills of infants and children have to be considered when attempting to assess neurological status. There is a tendency for ill children to regress to behaviour more befitting a younger child, especially if they are anxious or in pain. Therefore, effective pain control, empathy, and appropriate language are all essential factors when dealing with children. The presence of parents or other significant adults may help alleviate many communication difficulties, as well as helping to ease fear and anxiety and should therefore be encouraged.

A rapid assessment of the child's conscious level can be obtained by determining the AVPU score (Chapter 2) or by the Glasgow Coma Scale score if doctors and nurses are familiar with its use; there is a modified scale for children under five years of age. Additionally, assessing pupil size and reaction, the child's posture, muscle tone and any focal signs should be noted to determine neurological status.

Table 1.3   Blood pressure ranges by age systolic and mean

Blood pressure for age	1 month	1 year	5 years	10 years	15 years
50th centile for Systolic BP	75 mmHg	95 mmHg	100 mmHg	110 mmHg	120 mmHg
5th centile for Systolic BP	50 mmHg	70 mmHg	75 mmHg	80 mmHg	90 mmHg
50th centile for mean arterial pressure (MAP)	55 mmHg	70 mmHg	75 mmHg	75 mmHg	80 mmHg
5th centile for mean arterial blood pressure (MAP)	40 mmHg	50 mmHg	55 mmHg	55 mmHg	65 mmHg

E Exposure

To ensure that no significant clinical information is missed, examine the child fully by exposing their body. Appropriate measures to minimise heat loss (especially in infants) and respect dignity must be adopted at all times. The core body temperature should also be recorded, and if necessary, appropriate measures to normalise it initiated.

Weight estimation

Medications are prescribed based on a child's body weight. In an emergency situation, it is often impractical to weigh the child; therefore, an alternative method of estimating weight as accurately as possible is required. In order of preference:

1   Use the child/infant's body weight for drug calculations if known.

2   Use a body length tape with pre-calculated drug doses.

3   Use a paediatric emergency drug chart (Appendix A).

4   Use an age-based weight calculation formula. For the age group between one and ten years, the following formula provides an approximation of weight:

- Weight (kg) = (Age in years + 4) x 2.
- An infant weighs approximately 3 kg at birth and 10 kg at one year of age.

The simplicity of this formula facilitates recollection under pressure, and although the actual weight of overweight children will be underestimated, drug dosage is usually based on lean body mass rather than actual mass. For obese patients, use ideal body weight and do not use actual weight to avoid drug toxicity.

> Beware of exceeding the adult doses of drugs and fluids in older children (see Appendix A).

Whatever method is used to establish a child's bodyweight, all healthcare professionals must be prepared and sufficiently familiar in its use to be able to utilise it quickly and accurately.

Anticipatory care planning

A child may have a condition for which it is agreed that resuscitation would not be beneficial. Looking after such a child and their family requires compassionate and considered management (palliative care) and is beyond the scope of the PILS course.

In these circumstances, advance care planning is advocated, and RCUK supports the use of the ReSPECT (Recommended Summary Plan for Emergency Care and Treatment) process and form. This process is increasingly being adopted in hospitals throughout the UK, and all providers should be familiar with it.

It is important to feel that the best possible care has been delivered as not all resuscitation attempts are successful. Early intervention based on the ABCDE approach will reduce the number of unexpected deaths. The PILS course aims to provide this structured approach for the optimal care of children.

01: **Summary learning**

Children are more likely to suffer a secondary rather than a primary cardiorespiratory arrest.

Successful resuscitation from respiratory arrest, where there is still a cardiac output, is associated with 80–90% good quality, long-term survival.

Survival from full secondary cardiorespiratory arrest without neurological sequelae is considerably less likely (< 5% out of hospital and approximately 54% in hospital).

The respiratory and circulatory anatomy and physiology of infants and young children influence both the aetiology and the management of their illnesses/injuries.

The ABCDE approach is the basis of both the assessment and the management of seriously ill and/or injured children.

My key take-home messages from this chapter are:

Further reading

Atkins DL, Everson-Stewart S, Sears GK, Daya M, Osmond MH, Warden CR, Berg RA; Resuscitation Outcomes Consortium Investigators. Epidemiology and outcomes from out-of-hospital cardiac arrest in children: the Resuscitation Outcomes Consortium Epistry-Cardiac Arrest. Circulation 2009; 24;119:1484-91.

Naim MY, Burke RV, McNally BF et al. Association of Bystander Cardiopulmonary Resuscitation with Overall and Neurologically Favorable Survival after Pediatric Out-of-Hospital Cardiac Arrest in the United States; a report from the Cardiac Arrest Registry to Enhance Survival Surveillance Registry (CARES). JAMA Pediatr 2017;17(2):133-141.,

Haque IU, Zaritsky AL. Analysis for evidence for lower limit of systolic and mean arterial pressure in children, Paediatric critical care Medicine. 2007; 8, 2,138-122.

Office for National Statistics. Child and infant mortality in England and Wales (2018) (published February 2020) www.ons.gov.uk

www.respectprocess.org.uk

Litman RS, Weissend EE, Shibata D, Westesson PL. Developmental changes of laryngeal dimensions in unparalysed sedated children. Anesthesiology 2003:98:41-5.

Skellett S, Orzechowska I, Thomas K, Fortune PM. The landscape of paediatric in-hospital cardiac arrest in the United Kingdom National Cardia Arrest Audit. Resuscitation 2020;155:165-171.

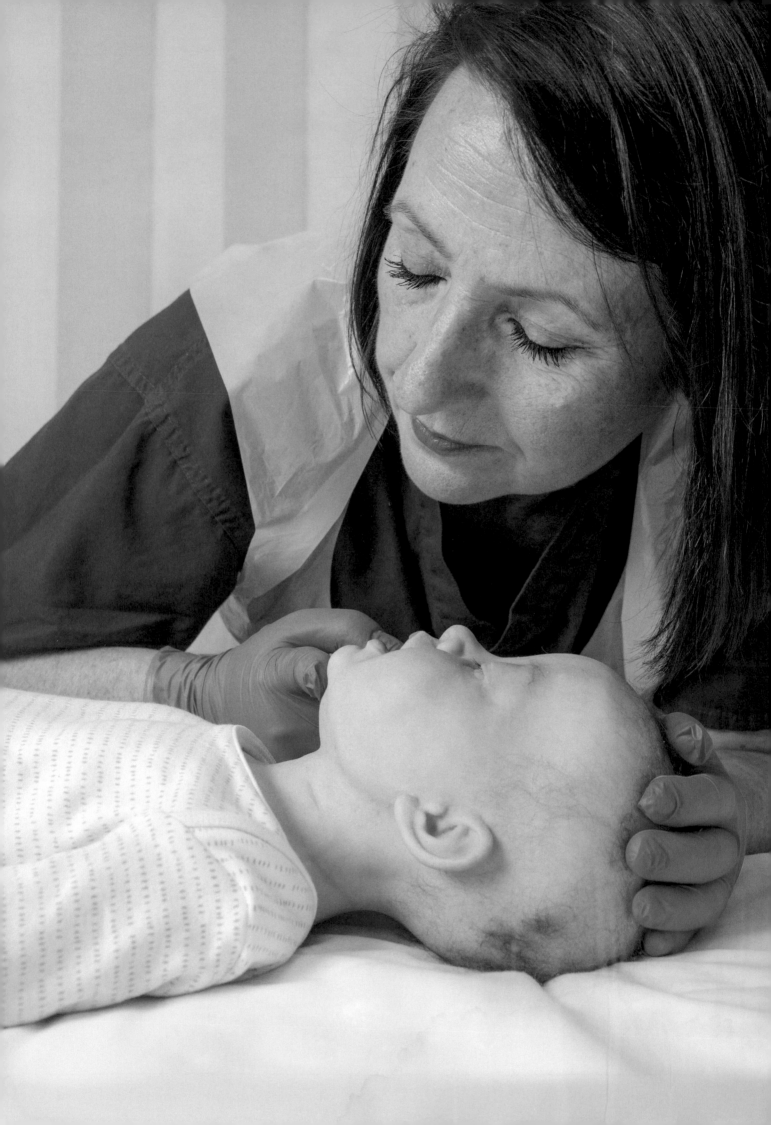

Recognition and initial management of the seriously ill child

02

Early recognition of the seriously ill child

In children, cardiorespiratory arrest is usually due to hypoxia, reflecting the end of the body's ability to compensate for the effects of underlying illness or injury. The initial problem may originate from the airway, breathing or circulation.

Irrespective of the primary aetiology, cardiorespiratory arrest in children is rarely a sudden event but a progressive deterioration from combined respiratory and circulatory failure. Early recognition and effective management of respiratory and/or circulatory failure will prevent the majority of paediatric cardiorespiratory arrests and thus reduce morbidity and mortality. It can also help identify children for whom attempted cardiorespiratory resuscitation may be inappropriate, which can help facilitate suitable end-of-life care.

The principles outlined in this chapter apply to the seriously ill child in all environments (i.e. the acute hospital setting or out-of-hospital). For some clinical settings, it is less common to see a critically ill child, and those responsible for the initial management might have limited experience. For all healthcare workers looking after the critically ill child, the structured ABCDE approach helps to ensure that potentially life-threatening problems are identified and managed in order of their priority.

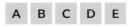

> Early recognition and effective management of respiratory and/or circulatory failure will prevent the majority of paediatric cardiorespiratory arrests and thus reduce morbidity and mortality

The A B C D E approach: general principles

1. Ensure personal safety and appropriate level of personal protective equipment.

2. Observe the child generally to determine the overall level of illness (i.e. do they look seriously unwell; are they interacting with parents/care providers). Speak to the child and assess the appropriateness of their response; ask the parents about the child's 'usual' behaviour and any concerns they have.

3. If they are unresponsive to your voice, administer tactile stimulation. If they respond by speaking or crying, this indicates that they have a patent airway, are breathing and have cerebral perfusion. Appropriate high-flow oxygen delivery should be commenced immediately.

4. Vital sign monitoring should be requested early (ECG, SpO$_2$ and non-invasive BP monitoring).

5. Circulatory access should be achieved as soon as possible. Blood test investigations and a bedside glucose estimation should be obtained.

6. Communicate findings of the ABCDE assessment to your team and other clinical and medical professionals called to help manage the patient. Outside of the intensive care unit, many hospitals employ an early warning score (EWS) system to aid in the detection of deteriorating children, and this information should also be highlighted. Structured communication tools such as SBAR (Situation, Background, Assessment and Recommendation) will aid the handover of important clinical information between teams (see Chapter 11).

7. Document your assessment and interventions as soon as possible.

A Airway problems

A review of practical airway management procedures is provided in Chapter 3.

Causes of upper airway obstruction

Airway obstruction can be partial or complete, sudden or insidious, progressive or recurrent. Respiratory rate and work of breathing generally increase in airway obstruction. When assessing airway patency, **chest movement does not guarantee that the airway is clear.** Air entry needs to be assessed as well by looking, listening and feeling for air movement and by chest auscultation.

Initially, airway obstruction is often partial but can lead to respiratory failure, exhaustion, secondary apnoea and eventually hypoxic brain damage. Additionally, partial airway obstruction can rapidly become total and result in cardiorespiratory arrest.

Congenital abnormalities such as choanal atresia or Pierre-Robin syndrome can be initially managed by the use of an appropriate airway adjunct to open the airway and buy time prior to definitive treatment.

Depression of the central nervous system can cause loss of airway control as protective upper airway reflexes and muscle tone are lost. This may be compounded in the infant due to the age-related anatomical features. In an unconscious infant, the pronounced occiput and short neck causes head flexion in the supine position and, together with the proportionately large tongue, this can quickly lead to airway obstruction.

Causes of central nervous system depression include hypoxia following decompensated respiratory or circulatory failure, head trauma, metabolic disorders (e.g. hypoglycaemia, inborn errors of metabolism), hypercapnia, alcohol and medications (e.g. opiates, benzodiazepines).

Airway obstruction due to these causes may not be accompanied by tachypnoea or increased work of breathing.

Recognition of upper airway obstruction

Airway obstruction may be demonstrated by difficulty in breathing and/or increased respiratory effort. In a conscious child, there may be visible distress. There may be additional respiratory noises, such as inspiratory stridor if the obstruction is partial. Causes are seen in Table 2.1.

Management of upper airway obstruction

The treatment of partial airway obstruction is to maintain airway patency and ensure that it does not become totally occluded. This may be achieved by head positioning, clearance of any secretions or foreign bodies, and summoning further assistance as indicated.

In patients with airway obstruction, delivery of supplemental oxygen is advised as early as possible to minimise the potential effects of hypoxia.

The conscious child will usually adopt a position that optimises airway patency. If the child is stable and deterioration is considered unlikely, they should be left with their parents/carers who can help administer oxygen and minimise stress and anxiety. Feeding should be avoided, and any fever treated to reduce increased metabolic demand. **If there is a decreased level of consciousness, airway compromise must be assumed.** The management priorities are to get more help whilst safeguarding the airway and preventing complications such as aspiration of gastric contents by placing the child in the recovery position or supporting the head-up position.

Basic airway opening manoeuvres (e.g. head tilt and chin lift or jaw thrust) should be used. Adjuncts such as oro/nasopharyngeal airways can also be used until more experienced help is available. Advanced emergency airway management may involve the insertion of a tracheal tube, supraglottic airway (e.g. i-gel, laryngeal mask airway (LMA)) or cricothyroidotomy, although the latter will only provide temporary oxygenation until a definitive airway can be achieved.

Table 2.1 Causes of airway obstruction

Causes of airway obstruction
Congenital abnormality (e.g. choanal atresia, Pierre-Robin syndrome)
Secretions (e.g. vomit, blood)
Respiratory tract infections (swelling or mucus secretions)
Pharyngeal swelling (e.g. oedema, infection)
Epiglottitis
Laryngotracheobronchitis (croup)
Nasal feeding tubes
Oxygen delivery devices (e.g. nasal cannulae)
Foreign body (e.g. food, toy, orthodontic appliances)
Central nervous system depression (loss of muscle tone)
Trauma (facial or throat)

B Breathing problems

In all seriously ill or injured children, the priority is for the appropriate management of the airway and ventilation (breathing).

Causes of breathing (respiratory) problems

Respiratory failure can result from acute or chronic breathing inadequacy. The underlying problem may be due to lung pathology (i.e. congenital or acquired diseases or trauma) or have a non-respiratory origin (e.g. circulatory failure, metabolic disorder, neurological problem).

The respiratory rate can be classified as abnormal if it is too rapid (tachypnoea), too slow (bradypnoea), or absent (apnoea). Respiratory distress is a clinical syndrome, which reflects increased work of breathing, often associated with attempts to increase tidal volume and can be associated with either tachypnoea or bradypnoea.

As the work of breathing increases, an increased proportion of the cardiac output is diverted to the respiratory muscles with a consequent increase in the amount of CO_2 produced.

Ultimately, if decompensation occurs, the respiratory system is unable to provide sufficient oxygen for tissue requirements, anaerobic metabolism occurs, and respiratory acidosis is complicated by metabolic acidosis.

Recognition of respiratory failure

From a physiological viewpoint, respiratory failure is usually defined as failure of the respiratory system to maintain an arterial oxygen level (PaO_2) > 9 kPa with 21% inspired O_2 (room air) and/or arterial carbon dioxide level of ($PaCO_2$) < 6.5 kPa. This definition requires arterial blood gas analysis.

PaO_2 of 9 kPa corresponds approximately to a peripheral oxygen saturation (SpO_2) of approximately 90%.

A child with respiratory distress may be able to maintain their arterial blood gas values within relatively normal limits by increasing their respiratory effort. Therefore, it is important to evaluate whether the child's situation is stable or if decompensation to respiratory failure is imminent. This evaluation requires knowledge of the signs and symptoms of respiratory distress and/or respiratory failure. When the compensatory mechanisms fail, deterioration is rapid and imminent cardiorespiratory arrest must be anticipated.

Warning signs are:

* decreased level of consciousness
* hypotonia (floppiness)
* decreased respiratory effort
* cyanosis or extreme pallor (despite oxygen being given)
* sweating
* bradycardia.

In children, recognition of respiratory failure is based on the full assessment of respiratory effort and efficacy, and the identification of evidence of respiratory inadequacy on major organs.

Work of breathing

Evidence of increased work of breathing is based on observation of the following:

- increased respiratory rate
- intercostal recession
- sternal recession
- subcostal recession
- use of accessory muscles (e.g. head bobbing)
- nasal flaring.

Respiratory rate

Tachypnoea is frequently the first indication of respiratory insufficiency. Normal respiratory rates vary with age, and this must be considered when determining the presence of tachypnoea (Table 2.2).

When referring to any chart with paediatric 'normal physiological values', be aware as none of these values taken in isolation has sufficient test performance and should always be considered in relation to other signs and symptoms.

Trends are more informative than single readings.

Changes in respiratory rate over time are very important. An increasing respiratory rate represents increasing physiological compensation to offset the deterioration in respiratory function. A sudden reduction in the respiratory rate in an acutely ill child is an ominous sign and may be a pre-terminal event. Causes may include exhaustion, central nervous system depression or hypothermia. Fatigue is always an important consideration in children; an infant with a respiratory rate of 80 min^{-1} will tire quickly.

Table 2.2   Respiratory rate ranges by age

Age (years)	Respiratory rate (breaths min^{-1})
< 1	30–40 min^{-1}
1–2	26–34 min^{-1}
2–5	24–30 min^{-1}
5–12	20–24 min^{-1}
> 12	12–20 min^{-1}

Recession

Recession (or retractions) may be sternal, subcostal or intercostal. The degree of recession gives an indication of the severity of respiratory disorder. Infants and young children can exhibit significant recession with relatively mild to moderate respiratory compromise, owing to their highly compliant chest wall. However, in children over approximately five years (by which age the chest wall is less compliant), recession is a sign of significant respiratory compromise.

Use of accessory muscles

When the work of breathing is increased, the sternocleidomastoid muscles in the neck are often used as accessory respiratory muscles. In infants, this may cause the head to bob up and down with each breath. This 'head bobbing' actually reduces the efficiency of each breath.

'See-saw' respiration

A breathing pattern, described as 'see-saw' respiration, is sometimes observed in severe respiratory compromise. It is the paradoxical movement of the abdomen during inspiration (i.e. the abdomen expands and the thorax retracts as the diaphragm contracts). This is inefficient respiration because the tidal volume is reduced, despite the increased muscular effort.

Inspiratory and expiratory noises

Normally, the airway above the thoracic inlet (extrathoracic) narrows and the airway below (intrathoracic) widens during the inspiratory phase of breathing. This pattern reverses on expiration. Observing the timing of an abnormal noise can indicate the site of airway obstruction. The presence of a high-pitched inspiratory noise (stridor) is characteristic of an upper airway (extrathoracic) obstruction and is due to rapid, turbulent flow through a narrowed portion of the upper tracheal airway. In severe obstruction, the stridor may also occur on expiration (biphasic stridor) but is usually less pronounced than it is during inspiration.

Wheezing is generally an expiratory noise. It is indicative of lower (intrathoracic) airway narrowing, usually at bronchiolar level, and maybe audible with the ear, or only on chest auscultation with a stethoscope.

The volume of airway noises is not indicative of the severity of respiratory compromise; diminishing noises may be indicative of increasing airway obstruction or exhaustion of the child.

Grunting

Grunting is mainly heard in neonates and small infants but can also occur in young children. It is the result of exhaling against a partially closed glottis and is an attempt to generate a positive end-expiratory pressure, thus preventing airway collapse at the end of expiration. Grunting is generally associated with 'stiff' lungs (e.g. respiratory distress syndrome, pulmonary oedema, atelectasis). Regardless of the underlying condition, grunting is an indication of severe respiratory compromise.

Nostril flaring

Flaring of the nostrils is often seen in infants and young children with increased respiratory effort.

Position

Children in respiratory distress will usually adopt a position to maximise their respiratory capacity. In upper airway obstruction, they often adopt a 'sniffing the morning air' position to optimise their upper airway patency. In generalised or lower respiratory problems, children often sit forward, supporting their weight on their arms, and holding on to (or wrapping their arms around) their knees. This position results in a degree of shoulder girdle 'splinting', which enhances accessory muscle use. The child should be supported in the position of optimal airway maximisation/comfort for them and have oxygen therapy given accordingly.

The degree of respiratory distress generally provides clinical evidence of the severity of respiratory insufficiency. However, there are three general exceptions to this (Table 2.3).

Table 2.3 Exceptions to increased work of breathing in respiratory failure

1. Exhaustion
Children who have had severe respiratory compromise for some time may have progressed to decompensation and no longer show signs of increased work of breathing. **Exhaustion is a pre-terminal event.**
2. Neuromuscular diseases
e.g. muscular dystrophy
3. Central respiratory depression
Reduced respiratory drive results in respiratory inadequacy (e.g. encephalopathy, medications such as morphine).

Efficacy of breathing

The infant's relatively higher metabolic rate and oxygen consumption accounts for their increased respiratory rates (Table 2.2). Thus, the effectiveness of breathing can be assessed by respiratory rate together with tidal volume, which in turn is evaluated by observation of chest movement, quality of cry, palpation, auscultation and percussion.

Additional information can be easily obtained by non-invasive pulse oximetry.

Chest movement, palpation and percussion

Observation of chest movement demonstrates the extent and symmetry of chest expansion. As well as revealing increased work of breathing, observing the movement of the chest wall can help identify diminished or asymmetrical respiratory effort.

Palpation of the chest wall may identify deformities, surgical emphysema or crepitus.

Percussion of the chest wall can demonstrate areas of collapse (dullness) or hyperresonance (e.g. in pneumothorax).

Chest auscultation

When listening with a stethoscope, air entry should be heard in all areas of the lungs. The volume of air movement occurring with inspiration and expiration can be estimated by auscultation. It is useful to compare the areas on one side of the chest with the other.

A very quiet or near-silent chest indicates a dangerously reduced tidal volume and is an ominous sign.

Pulse oximetry

A pulse oximeter should be used on any child with potential respiratory failure to provide an assessment of the patient's arterial oxygen saturation.

Without pulse oximetry, it is not always clinically possible to detect that the child has a decreased arterial oxygen saturation of haemoglobin (SaO_2) until the saturation is between 80–85%. Pulse oximetry is simple to use, relatively cheap, non-invasive and provides an immediate, objective measure of arterial blood oxygen saturation.

Start oxygen therapy if SpO_2 < 94% (or for infants or children with chronic conditions at an SpO_2 3% below known baseline). The goal is to keep the SpO_2 between 94–98% with as little supplemental oxygen as possible. When giving supplemental oxygen, sustained SpO_2 readings of 100% should generally be avoided (except in specific circumstances such as carbon monoxide poisoning). Do not give pre-emptive oxygen therapy to children and infants without signs of, or immediate risk of hypoxaemia or shock.

Pulse oximeter readings must not be used in isolation; it is vital to interpret them in light of the clinical picture and alongside other investigations and potential sources of error.

Pulse oximetry does not provide a reliable signal during CPR.

Effects of respiratory inadequacy on other body organs

Ongoing respiratory compromise rapidly affects other body organs/systems.

Heart rate

Hypoxia initially causes tachycardia. As this is a non-specific sign, it needs to be considered alongside other clinical signs. Severe or prolonged hypoxia ultimately leads to bradycardia, and therefore it is important to observe for trends rather than absolute values in heart rate. In a severely hypoxic child, bradycardia is a pre-terminal sign.

Skin perfusion

Hypoxia produces vasoconstriction and pallor of the skin. As their clinical condition deteriorates, the child's colour may become mottled before cyanosis appears centrally (lips and mouth). Cyanosis is not a reliable indicator of a degree of hypoxia; it may never be observed in the profoundly hypoxic child if there is significant anaemia. However, in a child with acute respiratory compromise, the development of central cyanosis is a late indication of severe hypoxia and is a pre-terminal sign.

Conscious level

Hypoxia and/or hypercapnia initially lead to agitation and/or drowsiness. Ongoing cerebral hypoxia ultimately results in loss of consciousness. In infants and young children, initial cerebral hypoxia may be difficult to detect, but their parents/carers frequently report that the infant/child is not responding to them as usual. This information is important and should not be ignored. The level of consciousness should be assessed using the AVPU score (Table 2.4).

Generalised hypotonia also accompanies cerebral hypoxia.

Table 2.4   The level of consciousness

A	Alert
V	responds to Voice
P	responds to Pain
U	Unresponsive to painful stimuli

The management of respiratory compromise

The initial treatment of breathing problems is dependent on achieving and maintaining a patent airway and effective delivery of oxygen. The method of oxygen administration will vary according to the child's clinical condition and age. Children who have adequate breathing should have high-flow oxygen delivered in a non-threatening manner and delivered in a way which is best tolerated by them (e.g. from a free-flow device held by their parents, a non-rebreathing face mask or nasal cannulae). When agitated the child's airflow will become turbulent and resistance to flow will increase.

In critically ill patients, those presenting with acute hypoxaemia or in the peri-arrest situation give high-concentration oxygen immediately. Give this initially with an oxygen mask with reservoir bag (non-rebreathing mask) using an oxygen flow of 12–15 L min⁻¹.

When breathing is inadequate (or absent), high-flow oxygen should be delivered by ventilation with a bag and mask system with a reservoir. In situations where the child is exhausted and is likely to need ongoing respiratory support, tracheal intubation may be indicated.

During cardiorespiratory arrest, use 100% oxygen to maximise arterial oxygen content and delivery to the tissues.

When the patient is stabilised, adjust the inspired oxygen concentration to maintain a SpO$_2$ of 94–98%. If pulse oximetry (with a reliable reading) is unavailable, continue oxygen via a reservoir mask until definitive monitoring or assessment of oxygenation is available.

C Circulatory problems

The appropriate management of the airway and ventilation (breathing) is the priority in all seriously ill children and should be addressed before considering their circulatory status.

Circulatory failure and shock

Shock is a clinical state where the delivery of oxygenated blood and associated nutrients (e.g. glucose) to the body tissues is inadequate for metabolic demand. Additionally, the removal of cellular waste (e.g. CO$_2$, lactic acid) may also be impaired.

Circulatory failure refers to insufficient blood being delivered to the body's tissues.

Shock may occur with increased, normal or decreased cardiac output (CO) or blood pressure (BP). Initially, the child's body can physiologically compensate for reduced tissue perfusion. However, when blood pressure starts to fall, as seen in circulatory failure, perfusion of the vital organs (e.g. brain, myocardium, kidneys) becomes increasingly compromised.

Compensated circulatory failure may have a normal blood pressure, but signs of abnormal perfusion: tachycardia, poor skin perfusion (prolonged capillary refill time), weak peripheral pulse, tachypnoea and reduced urine output.

Decompensated circulatory failure is present when hypotension develops, and vital organ perfusion is compromised. The clinical signs of inadequate tissue perfusion are much more apparent.

Aetiology of shock

Shock can arise from circulatory or respiratory failure. Most children with sustained shock, whatever its aetiology, have some degree of cardiovascular dysfunction requiring more than one type of treatment (i.e. managing the airway, breathing and circulation).

The most common causes of circulatory failure in children are hypovolaemia, sepsis or anaphylaxis.

Hypovolaemic shock: Characterised by decreased circulating volume (preload). It may result from severe fluid loss (as in dehydration) or haemorrhage.

Distributive shock: Typified by inadequate distribution of blood, so that the blood flow is insufficient for the metabolic demand of the tissues (e.g. anaphylaxis, sepsis or neurogenic).

Cardiogenic shock: Circulatory failure is less commonly the result of a primary cardiac problem due to congenital or acquired heart disease (e.g. cardiomyopathy, myocarditis or following cardiac surgery).

Obstructive shock: An uncommon cause of circulatory failure due to obstruction of blood flow to/from the heart (e.g. tension pneumothorax, cardiac tamponade or constrictive pericarditis).

Dissociative shock: Characterised by insufficient oxygen carrying capacity of the blood (e.g. anaemia or carbon monoxide poisoning).

Recognition of circulatory failure

In children, the recognition of circulatory failure is based on a complete cardiovascular assessment, looking for the effects of any circulatory insufficiency on major organs.

Parameters evaluated include:

- heart rate
- pulse volume
- capillary refill time
- blood pressure
- filling pressure (liver size in infants or jugular vein filling in older children)
- end-organ perfusion status.

Heart rate

The heart rate initially rises to maintain cardiac output.

Sinus tachycardia is a common response to many situations (e.g. pain, anxiety, fever), but it is also seen in hypoxia, hypercapnia and hypovolaemia. When tachycardia is accompanied by other signs of circulatory insufficiency, it is evidence of the body's attempts at physiological compensation. When the increased heart rate is unable to maintain adequate tissue perfusion, the tissue hypoxia and acidosis result in bradycardia.

The presence of bradycardia is a pre-terminal sign, indicating that cardiorespiratory arrest is imminent.

Pulse volume

Feeling for the volume (or amplitude) of central pulses (e.g. femoral, carotid, brachial) gives a subjective indication of stroke volume (SV); as SV decreases, so does the pulse amplitude. In progressive circulatory failure, the pulse amplitude diminishes, becomes weak and thready before finally, it is impalpable. Simultaneous palpation and comparison of central and peripheral pulses (e.g. radial and carotid) may be useful. Peripheral pulses decrease in amplitude earlier than central ones. Note that caution is required in their interpretation when vasoconstriction is present (e.g. ambient temperature is low, or in an anxious or pyrexial child).

The presence or absence of peripheral pulses is neither a specific nor a sensitive indicator of circulatory compromise but is useful in conjunction with other clinical signs.

However, diminishing central pulses are a pre-terminal sign, indicating that cardiorespiratory arrest is imminent.

Capillary refill and skin colour

The skin of a healthy child is warm to touch unless the ambient temperature is low. Their capillary refill time (CRT) is normally < 2 s, but when there is decreased skin perfusion, the CRT is prolonged. Be aware that CRT, although simple and quick to assess, is not very sensitive and like all observations, must not be assessed as a stand-alone observation. Evaluation of CRT is best performed by applying cutaneous pressure on the centre of the sternum for 5 s. Following removal of the pressure, the blanching of the skin should disappear within 2 s. A slower refill time (i.e. prolonged CRT) is indicative of poor skin perfusion. A pyrexial child with hypovolaemia will have a prolonged CRT, despite having a raised body temperature. A low ambient temperature or poor local lighting conditions reduces the accuracy of CRT. The CRT should be considered in context of the accompanying cardiovascular signs.

Initially, hypoxia produces vasoconstriction, and hence the child appears pale. As their clinical condition deteriorates, the child's colour becomes mottled and ultimately cyanosed. Cyanosis due to circulatory failure is initially peripheral, whereas hypoxaemia due to respiratory failure results in central cyanosis.

Peripheral vasoconstriction and decreased perfusion may also be indicated by a demarcation line between warm and cold skin. This can be detected by running the back of your hand up the child's limb. The demarcation line will travel towards the trunk over time if the child's condition is deteriorating, and vice versa if it is improving.

Table 2.5 Blood pressure ranges by age systolic and mean

Blood pressure for age	1 month	1 year	5 years	10 years	15 years
50th centile for Systolic BP	75 mmHg	95 mmHg	100 mmHg	110 mmHg	120 mmHg
5th centile for Systolic BP	50 mmHg	70 mmHg	75 mmHg	80 mmHg	90 mmHg
50th centile for mean arterial pressure (MAP)	55 mmHg	70 mmHg	75 mmHg	75 mmHg	80 mmHg
5th centile for mean arterial blood pressure (MAP)	40 mmHg	50 mmHg	55 mmHg	55 mmHg	65 mmHg

Blood pressure

In most forms of shock, the BP is initially maintained within the normal range (Table 2.5) for the child as a result of the body's compensatory mechanisms (e.g. tachycardia, vasoconstriction, increased myocardial contractility). Only when compensation is no longer possible does hypotension (BP less than 5th centile for age) occur, and a decompensated state results.

In hypovolaemia, approximately 40% of the child's total circulating volume can be lost before hypotension occurs. This means that BP only drops at a late stage in hypovolaemia (e.g. trauma, diarrhoeal illness, gut necrosis). It is therefore important that compensated circulatory failure is detected and managed at an early stage (i.e. before BP drops and decompensation occurs).

Table 2.5 shows the 5th and 50th centiles for systolic and mean BP for children. In full-term neonates, the lower limit for systolic BP (5th centile) is 50 mmHg, and for infants, from 1–12 months, it is 70 mmHg.

Regardless of the method used to obtain the BP (auscultatory or oscillometric) it is important that the appropriate cuff size is used. The cuff width should be > 80% of the child's upper arm length and the bladder should cover more than 40% of the circumference of their arm. The same size cuff should be used on each occasion that the BP is measured.

> Hypotension is a sign of physiological decompensation and indicates imminent cardiorespiratory arrest.

Filling pressure

If there is fluid overload, or if the heart is failing, the pressure in the veins supplying the heart is raised. This can be detected by listening for crackles at the lung bases, observing distention of the jugular veins in older children or feeling for enlargement of the liver in infants. If you are not able to assess this yourself, ask a suitably qualified team member to do this for you. Observation of these signs forms part of the reassessment following a fluid bolus.

Effects of circulatory inadequacy on other body organs

Ongoing circulatory compromise rapidly affects other body organs/systems:

Respiratory system

The metabolic acidosis that results from circulatory compromise leads to tachypnoea. However, there will not initially be other signs of increased work of breathing.

Conscious level

Hypoxia and/or hypercapnia initially lead to agitation and/or drowsiness. Progressive cerebral hypoxia ultimately results in loss of consciousness.

In infants and young children, initial cerebral hypoxia may be difficult to detect, but their parents/carers frequently report that the baby/child is not responding to them as usual and, as in respiratory failure, this information should not be ignored. The level of consciousness should be assessed by the AVPU score.

Generalised hypotonia also accompanies cerebral hypoxia.

Urine output

Information regarding the degree of reduced renal perfusion can be obtained by measuring the output of urine. A urinary output of < 2 mL kg^{-1} h^{-1} in infants or < 1 mL kg^{-1} h^{-1} in children older than one year is an indication of inadequate renal perfusion. Asking parents/carers about the child's urine output (e.g. the number of wet nappies; normal would be at least six wet nappies per day) may reveal a history of oliguria or anuria.

Management of circulatory compromise

The treatment of circulatory problems is dependent on achieving a patent airway and effectively managing ventilation with appropriate delivery of high-flow oxygen before turning attention to circulatory procedures.

Of course when there are immediately life-threatening causes of circulatory failure, such as massive or continuing haemorrhage, these must be managed simultaneously to managing A and B.

Insertion of at least one large-bore vascular cannula should be performed rapidly. This can be achieved by either intravenous or intraosseous routes.

In children with recognised shock, unless contraindicated (e.g. cardiac failure), volume replacement should be started with bolus therapy 10 mL kg^{-1} of balanced isotonic crystalloid solution (e.g. Plasma-Lyte, Ringer's Lactate, 0.9% sodium chloride). Glucose containing fluids with low sodium levels should NEVER be used for resuscitation; they should only be used to correct low blood glucose levels.

The use of vasoactive medications may be needed in fluid-resistant shock (circulatory access procedures, fluids and medications are in Chapter 6).

Cardiorespiratory failure

Signs of cardiorespiratory failure include alteration of consciousness, hypotonia, tachycardia, decreased central pulses and absent peripheral pulses. Bradycardia, hypotension, bradypnoea, gasping, and apnoea are terminal events preceding imminent cardiorespiratory arrest.

If any of the following signs are present, immediate intervention should be undertaken:

- coma or alteration of consciousness
- exhaustion
- cyanosis
- tachypnoea (RR > 60 min^{-1})
- HR < 100 min^{-1} for newborn
- HR > 180 min^{-1} or < 80 min^{-1} before one year (note: chest compressions in all ages should be started if HR < 60 min^{-1} with signs of inadequate perfusion)
- HR > 160 min^{-1} after one year
- seizures.

> A rapid assessment must be made of every child whom respiratory, circulatory or cardiorespiratory failure is expected.

D Disability – central neurological assessment

Following the appropriate management of the child's airway, ventilation and circulation, their neurological status should be evaluated.

Whilst both respiratory and circulatory failure can have central neurological effects, some neurological conditions may affect the respiratory and circulatory systems.

Neurological function

Conscious level

A rapid assessment of the child's conscious level can be determined by the AVPU score.

If required, a painful stimulus should be delivered either by applying pressure to the supraorbital ridge or rubbing the sternum. A child who is only responsive to painful (P)

Figure 2.1   Posturing   02

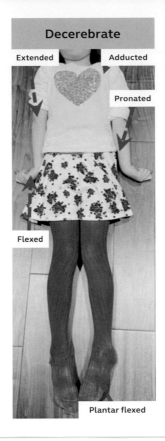
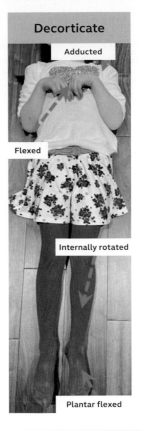

stimuli has a significant degree of neurological derangement equivalent to a Glasgow Coma Scale score of approximately 8.

Pupils

The size and reactivity of pupils can be affected by a number of things, including medications, intracranial pressure and cerebral lesions. Important signs to look for are dilatation, inequality and non-reactivity of the child's pupils. These features potentially indicate serious brain dysfunction.

Posture

Seriously ill children become hypotonic and floppy. However, if there is serious brain dysfunction, stiff posturing may be demonstrated. This posturing (which may only be evident when a painful stimulus is applied) can be decorticate (flexed arms and extended legs) or decerebrate (extended arms and legs); both indicate serious brain dysfunction and may be signs of raised intracranial pressure (Figure 2.1).

Blood glucose

Point of care blood sugar estimation should be performed in all seriously ill children. The increased metabolic rate associated with acute illness leads to increased use of glucose. Infants and small children do not have large glycogen liver stores, which can be broken down to generate more glucose and therefore may become hypoglycaemic with any acute illness, particularly when oral intake is reduced.

Specific assessments and actions in initial ABCDE approach

Assessment		Information sought	Possible resultant actions
On approaching the child		Note: • General appearance (colour, posture, activity) • Interaction with parent/caregiver	
A	Airway patency	Is the airway: • Patent (i.e. conscious, vocalising) • At risk • Obstructed	Suction if indicated Head positioning Oropharyngeal airway Reassess Summon expert help
B	Breathing adequacy	Note/observe/perform: • Conscious level • Air movement (look, listen, feel) • Respiratory rate • Chest expansion • Use of accessory muscles/recessions • Palpation • Percussion • Auscultation • SpO_2 and FiO_2	Administer high-flow oxygen appropriately Support breathing with bag-mask ventilation (BMV) as necessary Reassess Summon expert help
C	Circulation adequacy	Note/observe/perform: • Evidence of haemorrhage/fluid loss • Conscious level • Heart rate • Capillary refill time • Presence of distal/central pulses • Pulse volume features • Skin temperature and colour • Blood pressure • Urine output	Control any external bleeding Attach monitoring (as appropriate to setting) Obtain circulatory access (IV or IO) Estimate weight Blood samples for laboratory testing and bedside glucose estimation Fluid bolus (10 mL kg^{-1}) Reassess Summon expert help
D	Disability (conscious level)	Note: • AVPU score • Interaction with parent and surroundings • Posture and muscle tone • Pupil size and reactivity	Reconsider A, B and C management as conscious level dictates Establish bedside glucose estimation Establish if any medications have been given/possibly ingested Reassess Summon expert help
E	Exposure	Note/observe: • Evidence of any blood loss/skin lesions/wounds/drains/rashes etc. • Core temperature	Reconsider specific management e.g. antibiotics in sepsis Consider appropriate temperature control measures Reassess Summon expert help

Effects on other systems of central neurological failure

Central neurological dysfunction may affect other body systems.

Respiratory system

Comatose children with brain dysfunction may exhibit abnormal respiratory patterns (e.g. hyperventilation, Cheyne-Stoke respiratory pattern, alternate periods of hyperventilation and apnoea).

Circulatory system

Raised intracranial pressure causes the Cushing's triad (i.e. abnormal breathing pattern with bradycardia and hypertension). This is a late and pre-terminal sign of neurological failure.

Management of neurological compromise

The initial steps in the management of any child with a reduced conscious level must always be to maintain an open airway, ensure adequate ventilation and oxygenation, and support circulation in order to maintain cerebral oxygenation and perfusion.

Other causes of neurological compromise must then be considered, and specific investigations and treatments given as indicated (e.g. glucose for hypoglycaemia, CT scanning if head injury or cerebral infections are suspected).

E Exposure

To ensure that no additional significant clinical information is missed, record the child's temperature and examine the child fully by exposing their body (e.g. rashes). Appropriate measures to minimise heat loss (especially in infants) and respect dignity must be adopted at all times.

Further reading

Fleming S, Thompson M, Stevens R, et al. Normal ranges of heart rate and respiratory rate in children from birth to 18 years of age: a systematic review of observational studies. Lancet 2011;377:1011-8.

Plum F, Posner JB. The diagnostic of stupor and coma, 3rd edition. FA Davis Co, Philadelphia, USA, 1982.

Van de Louw A, Cracco C, Cerf C, et al. Accuracy of pulse oximetry in the intensive care unit. Intensive care medicine 2001;27:1606-13.

02: Summary learning

Early recognition of the seriously ill child prevents the majority of cardiorespiratory arrests, thus reducing morbidity and mortality.

The structured ABCDE approach helps ensure that potentially life-threatening problems are identified and dealt with in order of priority.

My key take-home messages from this chapter are:

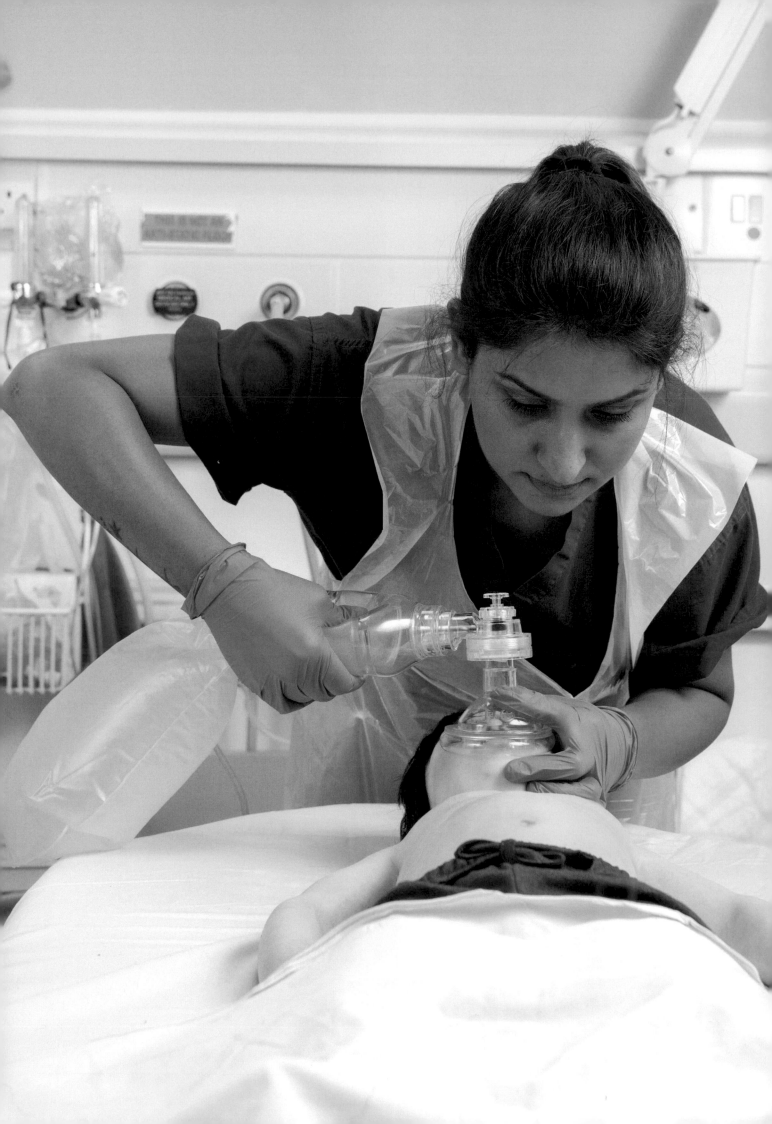

Management of the airway and ventilation

03

In this chapter

Airway management using positioning and adjuncts

Oxygen delivery devices

Assisted ventilation methods

Supraglottic airway (SGA) devices, intubation and capnography

The learning outcomes will enable you to:

Understand the causes and management of upper airway obstruction

Describe basic techniques to optimise the airway in initial resuscitation

Use simple adjuncts to assist in maintaining airway patency

Use simple devices for ventilation of the lungs

Causes of upper airway obstruction

Airway obstruction is a common occurrence in the seriously ill child. It may be the primary cause of the cardiorespiratory arrest (e.g. choking) or a consequence of the underlying disease process (e.g. seizures, head trauma), which leads to loss of consciousness.

In the unconscious child, the tongue can fall backwards and occlude their airway (Figure 3.1). Regardless of the cause, airway obstruction must be rapidly recognised and managed to prevent secondary hypoxic damage to the vital organs.

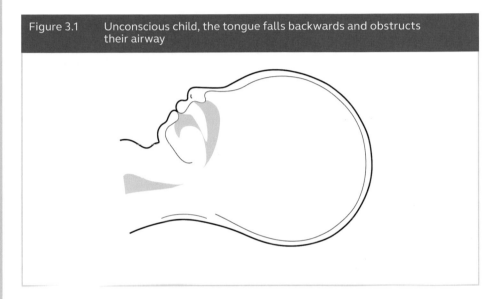

Figure 3.1   Unconscious child, the tongue falls backwards and obstructs their airway

Management of the airway and ventilation (breathing) is the first priority in dealing with the seriously ill child regardless of the underlying cause

Recognition of airway obstruction

In a conscious child, airway obstruction may be demonstrated by difficulty in breathing and/or increased respiratory effort. In both conscious and unconscious children, there may be additional respiratory noises if the obstruction is partial, whereas respiration will be silent if there is complete obstruction.

The most effective way to detect airway obstruction in all children is to look, listen and feel.

LOOK for chest (and abdominal) movements.

LISTEN for airflow at the mouth and nose (+/- additional noises).

FEEL for airflow at the mouth and nose.

LOOKING for breathing

During normal breathing the chest wall expands, and the abdomen is pushed slightly outwards as the diaphragm contracts. However, when the airway is obstructed, the abdomen protrudes markedly, and the chest is drawn inwards when the diaphragm contracts during inspiration ('see-saw' respiration). Additionally, accessory muscle usage and recession are likely to be observed. It can be difficult to differentiate these paradoxical movements from normal breathing, and the rescuer must also listen for the presence or absence of breath sounds and feel for air movement. If a clear face mask is being used, misting of the mask may be observed.

LISTENING for breathing

Normal respiration is quiet. Partially obstructed breathing is noisy, whilst completely obstructed breathing will be silent.

FEELING for breathing

The movement of air on inspiration and expiration can be felt at the mouth and nose (or tracheostomy) during normal breathing. If there is airway obstruction, this will be limited or absent.

Partial airway obstruction can quickly deteriorate to complete obstruction and therefore must always be considered as an emergency. Complete airway obstruction will lead to profound hypoxia, vital organ failure and cardiorespiratory arrest if the obstruction is not relieved very rapidly. Immediate action must be taken to relieve the obstruction and clear the airway.

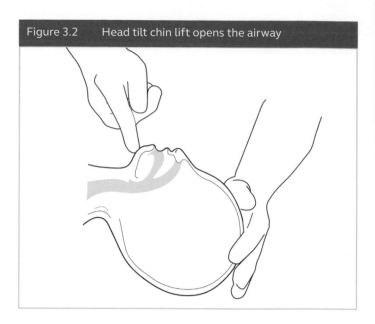

Figure 3.2   Head tilt chin lift opens the airway

Basic techniques to optimise the airway

Conscious children

If the child is making adequate spontaneous respiratory effort, they should be supported in a comfortable position (preferably the one they naturally assume themselves to optimise their airway). High-flow oxygen should be given in a manner that the child will tolerate whilst experienced help is sought.

Unconscious children

Whether or not the child is making spontaneous respiratory effort, the patency of the airway needs to be optimised immediately. This initially means positioning their head by performing either a head tilt and chin lift or a jaw thrust manoeuvre. Additionally, suction may be required to clear secretions, vomit or blood.

Head positioning

Open the child's airway by performing a head tilt and chin lift (Figure 3.2) or jaw thrust manoeuvre (Chapter 4). It is extremely important to ensure that head positioning techniques are carried out properly to make certain that neither hyperextension (Figure 3.3) nor excessive flexion of the neck occurs, as both will make obstruction worse. Take care not to compress the soft tissues under the child's jaw, as this can also occlude the airway.

Suction

Standard suction devices in hospitals are pipeline units. They consist of a wall terminal outlet, vacuum pressure regulator, a reservoir, tubing and a connector for an appropriate suction catheter to be attached.

In some low dependency hospital areas, during transportation and non-hospital environments such as GP surgeries, it is likely that the suction device available will be a portable device that is operated by battery or a hand/foot pump.

Large bore rigid suction catheters (e.g. Yankauer) are particularly useful for the clearance of thick or excessive

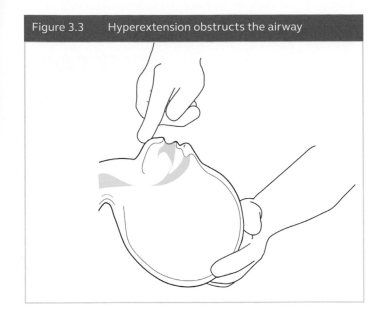

Figure 3.3   Hyperextension obstructs the airway

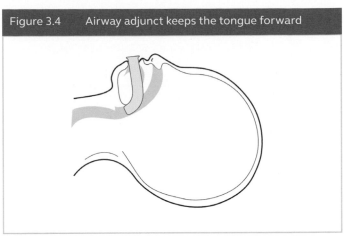

Figure 3.4   Airway adjunct keeps the tongue forward

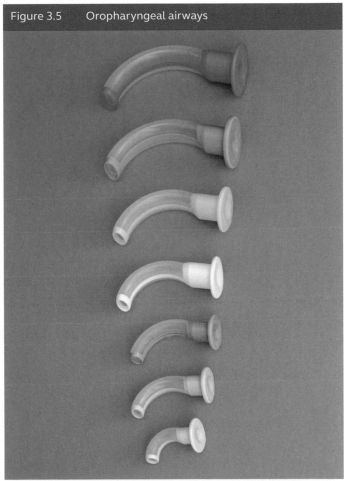

Figure 3.5   Oropharyngeal airways

secretions and vomit. Soft, flexible catheters in a range of sizes should also be available as these may be less traumatic to use and are particularly useful for nasal suction. They can also be passed through nasopharyngeal or oropharyngeal airways and tracheal tubes but they may not allow adequate clearance of thick or copious secretions.

Whichever suction catheter types are used, they should ideally have a side hole that can be occluded by the rescuer's finger to allow greater control over the suction pressure generated. Suction pressure should not exceed 120 mmHg in infants.

Airway suction must be carried out cautiously if the child has an intact gag reflex as it may induce vomiting, which can lead to aspiration or bradycardia.

Airway opening adjuncts

Oropharyngeal airways

The oropharyngeal airway (e.g. Guedel) is a rigid curved tube designed to open a channel between the lips and the base of the tongue (Figure 3.4). They are made of plastic and are reinforced and flanged at the proximal end. Practitioners should be aware that oropharyngeal airways colour coding and size classification are being standardised. Available sizes range from ISO 3.5 (previously labelled 000) for premature infants to ISO 10.0-12.0 (previously labelled 4–5) for large adults (Figure 3.5).

The correctly sized airway is one that, when laid against the side of the face, has a length equal to the distance between the level of the patient's incisors (or where they will be) to the angle of their jaw (Figure 3.6). If an incorrect size is used, it may result in trauma, laryngospasm and/or worsening of the airway obstruction.

The oropharyngeal airway should be inserted with great care using the minimum of force to avoid trauma and bleeding of the delicate palatal and pharyngeal mucosa. It is important to ensure that the tip of the oropharyngeal airway does not push the tongue back into the pharynx.

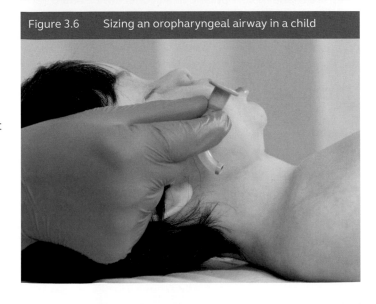

Figure 3.6   Sizing an oropharyngeal airway in a child

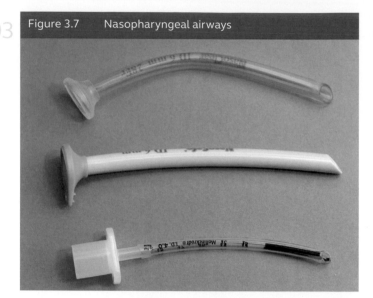

Figure 3.7   Nasopharyngeal airways

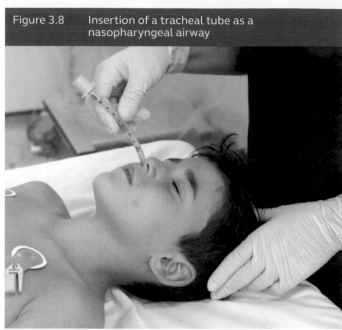

Figure 3.8   Insertion of a tracheal tube as a nasopharyngeal airway

The oropharyngeal airway can be introduced directly, sliding it carefully over the tongue, or alternatively, it can be introduced upside down initially and then rotated through 180° (this is the same technique as used in adults).

If this technique fails, a tongue depressor or laryngoscope blade can be used to open the oropharynx and introduce the airway directly.

Whichever technique is used, the effort required to insert the oropharyngeal airway should be minimal; do not use force.

Oropharyngeal airways are intended for use in unconscious patients. If the child is semi-conscious, they may cough, gag, vomit or develop laryngospasm. Insertion of the oropharyngeal airway should be abandoned if this occurs.

Following insertion of the oropharyngeal airway, the child's airway patency should be reassessed by the 'look, listen and feel' approach and oxygen given if indicated.

Nasopharyngeal airways

The nasopharyngeal airway is a flexible tube designed to open a channel between the nostril and the nasopharynx. They are made of soft plastic or silicone, are bevelled at the insertion end and flanged at the outer end (Figure 3.7). The flange prevents the airway from passing completely into the nasal passage. Tracheal tubes cut to the correct length may alternatively be used (Figure 3.8)

The correct insertion depth should be sized from the nostrils to the tragus of the ear. An appropriate tube size can be estimated by matching its diameter against the diameter of the child's anterior nares, and when inserted, it should not cause blanching of the nostril.

Once appropriately sized, the nasopharyngeal airway should be lubricated and introduced into the nostril. With a gentle rotating motion, the airway should be passed directly backwards and posteriorly along the

floor of the nostril. The tube should not be directed upwards as this will cause trauma and bleeding. Following insertion of the nasopharyngeal airway, the child's airway patency should be reassessed by the 'look, listen and feel' approach and oxygen given if indicated.

Nasopharyngeal airways may be better tolerated by conscious children than oropharyngeal airways and are useful as adjuncts in the management of children who may improve their level of consciousness (e.g. the fitting child who is becoming less obtunded).

Their use is contraindicated in patients where basal skull fracture is suspected or if there is a coagulopathy.

Oxygen delivery and ventilatory support

Oxygen should be given as soon as it is available. Initially, this should be at the highest available concentration for all seriously ill children; concerns about oxygen toxicity should never prevent its use during resuscitation. Oxygen should be regulated using a flowmeter capable of delivering up to 15 L min^{-1} (although this may be much higher when high-flow nasal cannulae are used via a special flowmeter). It should ideally be warmed and humidified to minimise the risks of airway irritation and hypothermia. The method used to deliver the oxygen should be selected according to the child's clinical condition. Oxygen saturation levels should be monitored by pulse oximetry (SpO$_2$). When the child's condition has stabilised, the inspired oxygen concentration should be reduced whilst monitoring SpO$_2$ to maintain adequate oxygenation.

Oxygen concentration can be expressed as a % or as the fraction of inspired oxygen FiO$_2$ (where 100% oxygen is the equivalent to an FiO$_2$ of 1.0). Table 3.1 shows the amount of oxygen that is delivered for each oxygen delivery device.

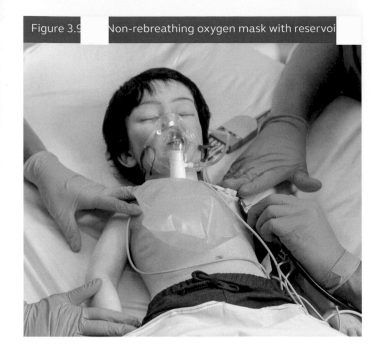

Figure 3.9   Non-rebreathing oxygen mask with reservoir

When the side valves (or flaps) over the inspiratory holes are removed, a lower FiO_2 will be achieved, as room air will be drawn into the mask as the child inhales.

Simple oxygen mask

A simple oxygen mask without a reservoir bag can deliver oxygen concentrations of up to 60% at flow rates of 10–15 L min⁻¹. Room air is entrained around the edges of the mask and through the holes in the mask so diluting the oxygen delivery.

'Blow-by' facial oxygen

Either the end of the oxygen tubing or a face mask can be held by the child's carer at a short distance from the child's face. This is a less threatening method that can help to alleviate the child's fear and maximise their cooperation. However, the inspired concentration that can be delivered is low and inconsistent, so it is only suitable for children with mild respiratory compromise who cannot tolerate other methods of oxygen delivery. Oxygen flow rates need to be adjusted depending on what the child will accept.

Nasal cannulae

This method can be useful in stable children of all ages, particularly in pre-school children. The delivery of oxygen via cannulae (or 'prongs') is dependent on oxygen flow and nasal resistance, but the FiO_2 will be low and variable, so it is not suitable during a resuscitation or when a high oxygen concentration is required. They are also not suitable for use in children with copious or tenacious nasal secretions, as they will easily become blocked. Flow rates should be kept below 4 L min⁻¹ as higher flows are extremely irritating to the nasal passages and do not significantly increase oxygen delivery.

High-flow nasal cannula oxygen (HFNC)

Heated, humidified, high-flow nasal cannula oxygen (e.g. Optiflow, Vapotherm) is increasingly being used for critically ill patients, as it has the advantage of humidifying and warming gases. It is also able to deliver a higher FiO_2 (up to 1.0) than standard nasal cannulae. At high oxygen flow rates, HFNC is able to increase functional residual capacity, improve mucociliary clearance of secretions and also probably deliver some positive end-expiratory pressure (PEEP) which can be advantageous for hypoxic children (e.g. pneumonia, pulmonary contusion, and bronchiolitis). Flows of 2 L kg⁻¹ min⁻¹ are commonly used for children up to 12 kg, plus 0.5 L kg⁻¹ min⁻¹ for each kg thereafter to a maximum of 50 L min⁻¹.

Table 3.1   Oxygen delivery devices, flow rates and maximum inspired oxygen levels

Device	Flow rate	Maximum inspired
Nasal prongs	Maximum 4 L min⁻¹	40%
Oxygen mask without reservoir	10–15 L min⁻¹	60%
Oxygen mask with reservoir	Must be enough to avoid reservoir collapse during inspiration, e.g. 12–15 L min⁻¹	90%
Humidified High-flow nasal cannulae (HFNC)	4–50 L min⁻¹*	100%

*Will vary between manufacturers

Oxygen administration methods

Oxygen mask with reservoir bag

This is the preferred method for delivering oxygen to a seriously ill child who is breathing spontaneously. The flow of oxygen must be sufficiently high to ensure the reservoir bag fills adequately (Figure 3.9). It is possible to give an oxygen concentration up to 90% with an oxygen delivery flow of 12–15 L min⁻¹.

These devices have three 'one-way' valves; one between the reservoir bag and the mask and one on each side of the face mask over the inspiratory holes. They are designed so that when the child inhales, the valve between the mask and reservoir bag opens, allowing oxygen to flow into the mask, whilst those on the either side of the mask close to prevent in-drawing of room air. When the child exhales, the valve between the mask and reservoir bag closes whilst the ones on either side of the mask open to allow the escape of the child's expired breath (i.e. there is no rebreathing of gas).

Methods of assisted ventilation

If a child stops breathing completely or if spontaneous ventilation is inadequate, positive pressure ventilatory support is required.

When providing positive pressure ventilation for an infant/child, aim for a respiratory rate of 12–30 min^{-1} with younger children having higher rates. The volume delivered should be sufficient to produce a normal visible chest expansion, and breath sounds on auscultation. Lower rates of ventilation are used for children and infants who have an advanced airway in place during cardiorespiratory arrest (see Chapter 9).

Continuous monitoring of the heart rate and SpO_2 should be undertaken as soon as practicable.

Mouth-to-mask devices

The pocket mask is widely used in resuscitation of apnoeic adults, and the standard size may be suitable for use in larger children and adolescents. There is a 'paediatric' pocket mask available, but "one size" does not fit all infants and children, and an appropriate size of paediatric face mask may need to be substituted. Expired air ventilation using a pocket mask should only be used if a manual ventilation device (e.g. self-inflating bag system) is not immediately available.

When it is deemed appropriate for use (e.g. in an adolescent), the pocket mask is a device designed to minimise infection risks when delivering expired air ventilation. The device is made of transparent plastic with a one-way valve that directs the patient's expired breath away from the rescuer. An oxygen delivery port (which also has a one-way valve) is incorporated into some pocket masks and allows supplemental oxygen to be administered.

Technique for mouth-to-mask ventilation:

- Having assembled the pocket mask, the rescuer positions themselves behind the supine child.
- The child's head should be placed in an appropriate position (e.g. 'sniffing' position) to achieve a patent airway.
- Apply the mask over the child's mouth and nose, pressing down with the thumbs of both hands to create a seal.
- Lift the child's jaw upwards (jaw thrust) into the mask with the other fingers, taking care not to compress the soft tissues under the mandible.
- Blow through the mask's one-way valve until chest expansion is observed (Figure 3.10).
- Stop inflation and observe the chest falling.
- Repeat as appropriate.

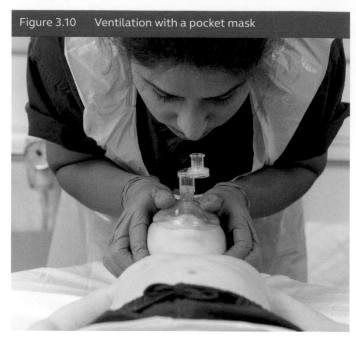

Figure 3.10   Ventilation with a pocket mask

- If chest expansion is not seen, assess whether this may be due to inadequate airway patency or a poor seal between the child's face and the mask, and correct as necessary.
- If the mask has an appropriate port and there is oxygen available, supplemental oxygen should be administered.

This technique can also be used with a standard face mask, but it will not provide protection against infection unless a breathing system filter is also used.

The self-inflating bag device (as used for bag-mask ventilation)

In a child who has inadequate/absent breathing, maintenance of a patent airway is the first priority of management. Once this is achieved, adequate ventilation must be established. A self-inflating bag can be connected to a face mask, tracheal tube, or SGA when these are in place. Self-inflating bags can be used with or without a supplemental oxygen source. However, in cardiopulmonary resuscitation situations, oxygen is almost always used in order to deliver ventilation with a high inspired oxygen concentration.

A self-inflating bag system consists of a bag that the operator squeezes to deliver a breath to the patient. Exhalation occurs through a one-way valve at the patient end of the bag, whilst the device automatically refills with air (and oxygen when attached) via an inlet at the opposite end.

Used without supplemental oxygen, a self-inflating bag system will ventilate with room air (21% oxygen). The oxygen concentration can be increased to approximately 50% by attaching a high-flow of oxygen to the oxygen port on the base of the bag, without a reservoir bag. As described above, the use of the reservoir bag, together with high-flow of oxygen at 15 L min^{-1}, will enable the delivery of > 90% oxygen (Figure 3.11).

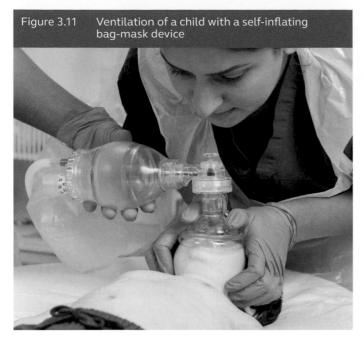

Figure 3.11   Ventilation of a child with a self-inflating bag-mask device

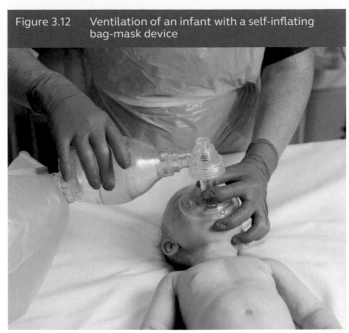

Figure 3.12   Ventilation of an infant with a self-inflating bag-mask device

Self-inflating bags are available in three or four sizes, depending on the manufacturer (e.g., 250, 450–500, 900–1200 and 1600–2000 mL). Smaller sizes usually have a pressure-limiting valve that prevents excessive inflation pressures that otherwise may cause barotrauma. The pressure limit is pre-determined by the manufacturers (usually 30–40 cm H_2O). During cardiopulmonary resuscitation, higher than normal inflation pressures may be required, and the pressure limiting valve may need to be overridden. The most common reason for needing to activate the pressure-limiting valve is upper airway obstruction due to a poor airway opening technique. Thus, ensure that the child's airway is patent (e.g. check head positioning) before overriding the valve. It should be noted that such valves are now being incorporated into some of the large bag sizes.

The smallest bags (approximately 250 mL) are intended for use in preterm neonates < 2.5 kg only. They are not appropriate for use in full-term neonates and infants as they may be inadequate to support effective tidal volume. When selecting the bag size, rescuers should follow manufacturers' guidance for age and weight ranges. The bag volume should always be able to support sufficient tidal volume for the patient. Regardless of size, the provider should only use the force and tidal volume necessary to cause visible chest expansion (Figures 3.11, 3.12).

Self-inflating bags should not be used to deliver oxygen to spontaneously breathing patients. Depending on the valve system, this may result in the inspiration of room air (or even rebreathing of the child's own passively expired air if the mask is held tightly on the face) as the child's own respiratory efforts may not generate sufficient pressure to open the valve. Children who are making an adequate respiratory effort should therefore have oxygen administered by another method.

Face mask selection

These are the interface between the ventilation device and the child. They must be capable of providing a good seal over the mouth and nose whilst ensuring minimal pressure is applied over the eyes.

Masks are available in a variety of sizes and two basic types; anatomically shaped ones for older children and adults and circular ones for infants and small children (Figure 3.13). The preferred mask is transparent (to allow rapid detection of secretions/vomit and observation of the child's central colour) and should have a low dead space.

Correctly performed BMV is an important skill for all healthcare professionals who work with children. Whilst the operating principle of self-inflating bags is simple, they require skill and practice to use them safely and effectively.

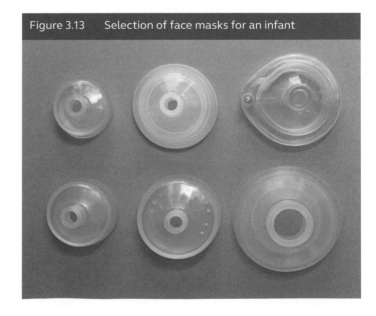

Figure 3.13   Selection of face masks for an infant

Hypoventilation can occur with poor technique (e.g. inadequate mask seal or incorrect head positioning) and is likely to have a negative effect on the outcome.

Excessive ventilation volume can distend the stomach, which reduces ventilation and increases the risk of gastro-oesophageal reflux and aspiration.

When self-inflating bags are used with a face mask, it can be difficult for a single rescuer to achieve an airtight seal whilst simultaneously using one hand to maintain a patent airway with a jaw thrust manoeuvre and squeezing the bag with the other. A two-person technique (one person to maintain the airway and hold the mask in position, and the second to squeeze the bag) will usually overcome these difficulties and is the recommended technique in resuscitation (Figure 3.11).

Technique for bag-mask ventilation (two-person technique):

- Having selected the appropriate size of bag and mask, one rescuer should stand behind the supine child.

- The oxygen supply should be connected at a high-flow and the reservoir bag should be seen to inflate.

- A second person should stand slightly to one side of the child's head.

- The child's head should be placed in an appropriate position (e.g. 'neutral' position for an infant, 'sniffing the morning air' in the older child) to achieve a patent airway. A roll placed under the infant's shoulders is often useful to assist in maintaining an appropriate airway position (unless contraindicated in trauma cases).

- The first rescuer applies the mask over the child's mouth and nose, gently pressing down with the thumb and index finger of both hands. Then lift the child's jaw upwards (jaw thrust) into the mask with the other fingers, with one finger under the angle of the jaw. Take care not to compress the soft tissues underneath the mandible.

- The second rescuer gently squeezes the bag until normal chest expansion is observed.

- Stop inflation and observe the chest falling.

- Repeat as appropriate.

- If chest expansion is not seen, assess whether this may be due to inadequate airway patency or a poor seal between the child's face and the mask, and correct as necessary.

Bag-mask ventilation frequently results in gastric distension, and therefore the placement of a gastric tube should be undertaken as early as practicable.

T-piece (flow-inflating bag) circuit

This equipment is often employed by anaesthesia and critical care staff. It requires a continuous gas source for inflation of the bag, and therefore there must always be an appropriate self-inflating system immediately available in case there is a failure of the gas supply. The safe and effective use of this equipment requires considerable expertise, and it should be utilised by experienced practitioners only.

Supraglottic airway devices

There are several SGAs that have been used successfully in children under anaesthesia. They may also be useful in resuscitation. These include the laryngeal mask airway and i-gel and are designed to sit above the glottis and may provide an effective airway to achieve ventilation and oxygenation.

Trained providers could consider SGA insertion if BMV is difficult or not successful (Figure 3.14).

Tracheal intubation

Tracheal intubation should only be performed by experienced personnel who have been trained to perform the technique.

The indications for and the techniques associated with tracheal intubation are beyond the scope of the PILS course. The most important ventilation skill required of healthcare professionals dealing with children is effective BMV with a self-inflating bag device. The vast majority of children can be safely managed with BMV until expert help is available.

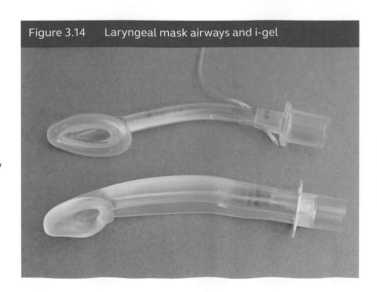

Figure 3.14   Laryngeal mask airways and i-gel

03: Summary learning

Airway management is the first priority in the care of the critically ill or injured child and is central to successful paediatric resuscitation.

The delivery of high-flow oxygen with the use of simple airway manoeuvres and BMV provides effective first-line management in the critically ill child.

SGA devices and tracheal intubation is reserved for those experienced in the technique.

My key take-home messages from this chapter are:

Further reading

Blevin AE, McDouall SF, Rechner JA, Saunders TA, Barber VS, Young JD, Mason DG. A comparison of the laryngeal mask airway with the facemask and oropharyngeal airway for manual ventilation by first responders in children. Anaesthesia. 2009;64:1312-6.

Bhende MS, Thompson AE. Evaluation of an end tidal carbon dioxide detector during pediatric cardiopulmonary resuscitation. Pediatrics 1995; 95:395-399.

De Caen AR, Kleinman ME et al. Part 10: Pediatric basic and advanced life support 2010 International Consensus on Cardiopulmonary Resuscitation and Cardiovascular Care Science with Treatment Recommendations. Resuscitation 2010;81s:e213-259.

Johnson M, Miskovic A, Ray S et al. The nasopharyngeal airway: Estimation of the nares-to-mandible and nares-to-tragus distance in young children to assess current clinical practice. Resuscitation 2019;140:50-54

Ellis DY, et al. Cricoid pressure in emergency department rapid sequence tracheal intubations: a risk-benefit analysis. Ann Emerg Med 2007;50:653-65.

Gausche M, Lewis RJ, Stratton SJ, et al. Effect of out-of-hospital pediatric endotracheal intubation on survival and neurological outcome: a controlled clinical trial. JAMA 2000;283:783-90.

Eich C, Roessler M, Nemeth M, Russo SG, Heuer JF, Timmermann A. Characteristics and outcome of prehospital paediatric tracheal intubation attended by anaesthesia-trained emergency physicians. Resuscitation 2009;80:1371 7.

Ghai B, Wig J. Comparison of different techniques of laryngeal mask placement in children. Curr opin Anesth 2009; 22:4000-404.

Grein AJ, Weiner GM. Laryngeal mask airway versus bag-mask ventilation or endotracheal intubation for neonatal resuscitation. Cochrane Database Systemic Review 2005; CD003314. www2.cochrane.org/reviews/en/ab003314

Kwon, JH, et al. Analysis of the functionally-narrowest portion of the pediatric upper airway in sedated children. Medicine, 2018; 97;27:, e11365. https://doi.org/10.1097/MD.0000000000011365

Warner KJ, et al. Prehospital management of the difficult airway: a prospective cohort study. J Emerg Med 2009;36:257-65.

Weiss M, Dullenkopf A, Fischer JE, Keller C, Gerber AC European Paediatric Endotracheal Intubation Study Group. Prospective randomised controlled multi-centre trial of cuffed or uncuffed endotracheal tubes in small children. Br J Anaesth. 2009;103:867-73.

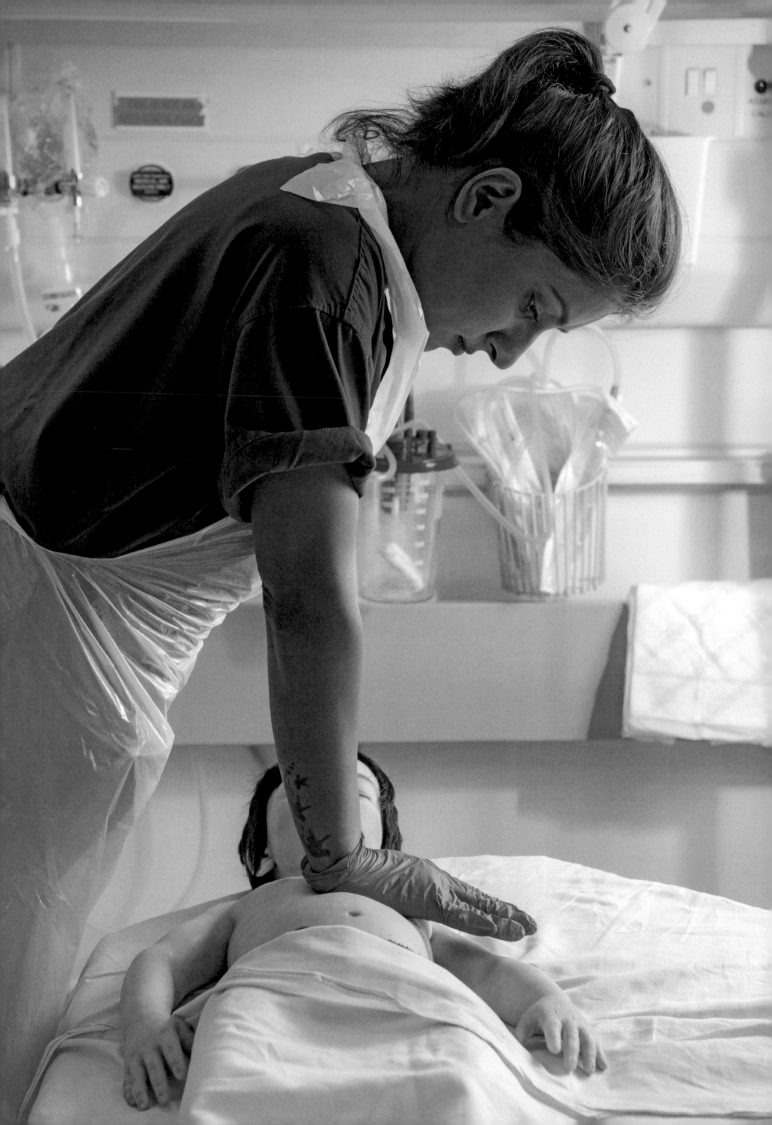

Basic life support

In this chapter

Age definitions

Infant and child basic life support sequence

Recognition and management of choking

Recovery positions

The learning outcomes will enable you to:

Understand the importance of early effective basic life support (BLS) for decreasing mortality and morbidity

Describe how and when to activate the Emergency Medical Service (EMS) or the in-hospital clinical emergency team

Understand the rationale for the sequence of steps in BLS both in and out of hospital

Consider the importance of early appropriate choking management

Understand the rationale for the different techniques of BLS employed in infants and children

Introduction

BLS is the combination of manoeuvres and skills that, without technical adjuncts, provides recognition and management of a person in cardiac or respiratory arrest and 'buys time' until the individual can receive more advanced treatment. BLS must be started as rapidly as possible. Its main objective is to achieve sufficient oxygenation and perfusion to 'protect' the brain and other vital organs. Ideally, all citizens should possess BLS knowledge and skills. The sequence of actions in BLS is known as cardiopulmonary resuscitation (CPR).

Age definitions

For the purposes of basic life support (BLS), an infant is a child less than one year excluding newborn, and a child is aged between one year and 18 years. The differences between adult and paediatric resuscitation are largely based on different aetiology; studies have shown that the paediatric causes of cardiorespiratory arrest continue into early adulthood. If the rescuer believes the individual to be a child, then they should use the paediatric guidelines.

Background

In the management of the collapsed child, a number of factors are critical in maximising the chances of a good outcome. The most important is the early recognition and appropriate intervention in children who exhibit signs of respiratory and/or circulatory compromise. Prevention of cardiorespiratory arrest by the optimal management of respiratory distress and/or circulatory failure will improve the prognosis (Chapters 1 and 2).

Nevertheless, there will always be some children in whom respiratory and/or circulatory collapse cannot be prevented. For these children, early BLS, rapid activation of the Emergency Medical Service (EMS) or in-hospital clinical emergency team and prompt, effective, advanced life support are crucial in improving mortality and morbidity.

Basic life support must be started as rapidly as possible

BLS sequence

Although unusual, a primary cardiac arrest does occasionally occur in children. If this situation is likely, such as a sudden, witnessed collapse of a child with a known cardiac condition, optimal outcome will depend on early defibrillation. It is then preferable for a lone rescuer to activate the EMS before starting BLS and to use an automated external defibrillator (AED), if available.

However, for the majority of children who suffer cardiorespiratory arrest, the recommended sequence of events is based on two facts:

- Cardiorespiratory arrest is hypoxic in origin, and therefore the priority is prompt oxygenation provided by rescue breaths or bag-mask ventilation (BMV).

- The most common cardiac arrhythmia is profound bradycardia deteriorating into asystole; hence effective BLS is more important than access to a defibrillator.

The sequence of actions in paediatric BLS will depend upon the level of training of the rescuer attending:

- Healthcare professionals with a duty to respond to paediatric emergencies should be fully competent in paediatric BLS as they have an obligation to deliver more comprehensive care; this specific sequence is detailed later in this chapter (Figure 4.13).

- Those trained only in 'adult' BLS (may include healthcare providers and lay rescuers) who have no specific knowledge of paediatric resuscitation should use the adult sequence they are familiar with, including paediatric modifications (Figure 4.1).

- Bystander CPR should be started in all cases when feasible. The EMS dispatcher has a crucial role in assisting lay untrained bystanders to recognise cardiorespiratory arrest and provide CPR. When bystander CPR is already in progress at the time of the call, dispatchers may only provide instructions when asked for or when issues with knowledge or skills are identified.

- It is important that rescuers follow the specific order of steps in BLS because if one manoeuvre is missed or incorrectly performed, the effectiveness of the next step is likely to also be compromised, hence the order of delivering the resuscitation sequence: Airway (A), Breathing (B) and Circulation (C).

- BLS is more effective when the rescuer is proficient in its delivery, but even suboptimal CPR gives a better result than no CPR at all. Hence rescuers unable or unwilling to provide mouth to mouth ventilation should be encouraged to perform at least compression-only CPR. A child or infant is far more likely to be harmed if the bystander does nothing.

Out-of-hospital BLS (with paediatric modifications)

S	Safety
S	Stimulate
S	Shout for assistance
A	Airway
B	Breathing
C	Circulation

S – Safety

In all emergencies, quickly assess the situation and ensure the safety of first the rescuer(s) and then that of the child; although the potential hazards may be different, this is equally important whether the situation occurs within or outside the healthcare environment.

All bodily fluids should be treated as potentially infectious; put on gloves as soon as practicable and use barrier devices for ventilation (e.g. pocket mask) if possible. Whilst the efficacy of face shields is uncertain, and they may not reliably prevent transmission of infection, their use affords some protection and may make it more acceptable for the receipt or delivery of rescue breaths.

On approaching the child, and before touching them, rapidly look for any clues as to what may have caused the emergency as this may influence the way the child is managed (e.g. any suspicion of head or neck injury necessitates consideration of cervical spine immobilisation).

S – Stimulate

It is important to establish the responsiveness of the apparently unconscious child by tactile and verbal stimulation as they may not be in a critical condition. You can do this by stabilising the child's head by placing one hand on their forehead and then tugging their hair whilst calling their name or telling them to "wake up". Never shake a child vigorously.

If the child responds (e.g. moves, cries or talks):

- leave the child in the position in which you find them (provided they are not in further danger)

- check their condition and get help if needed

- reassess the child regularly.

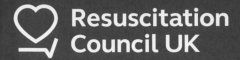
Paediatric out-of-hospital basic life support

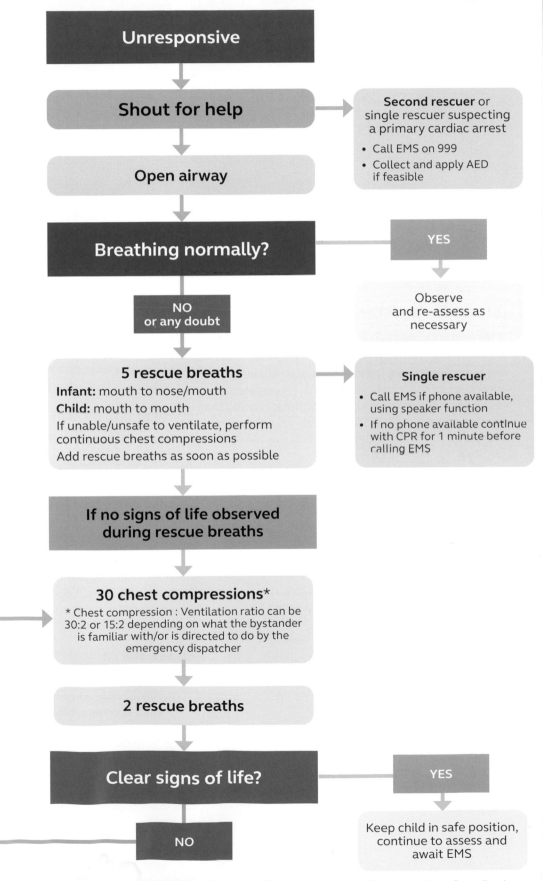

Unresponsive

Shout for help

Second rescuer or single rescuer suspecting a primary cardiac arrest
- Call EMS on 999
- Collect and apply AED if feasible

Open airway

Breathing normally?

YES → Observe and re-assess as necessary

NO or any doubt

5 rescue breaths
Infant: mouth to nose/mouth
Child: mouth to mouth
If unable/unsafe to ventilate, perform continuous chest compressions
Add rescue breaths as soon as possible

Single rescuer
- Call EMS if phone available, using speaker function
- If no phone available continue with CPR for 1 minute before calling EMS

If no signs of life observed during rescue breaths

30 chest compressions*
* Chest compression : Ventilation ratio can be 30:2 or 15:2 depending on what the bystander is familiar with/or is directed to do by the emergency dispatcher

2 rescue breaths

Clear signs of life?

YES → Keep child in safe position, continue to assess and await EMS

NO

Those trained only in 'adult' BLS (may include healthcare providers and lay rescuers) who have no specific knowledge of paediatric resuscitation, should use the adult sequence they are familiar with, including paediatric modifications.

Figure 4.1   Paediatric out-of-hospital basic life support

41

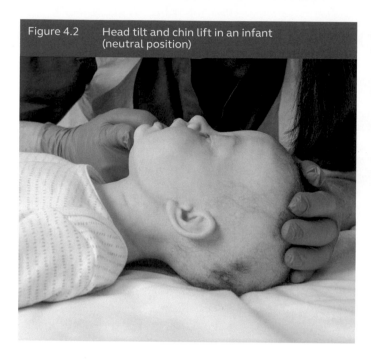

Figure 4.2   Head tilt and chin lift in an infant (neutral position)

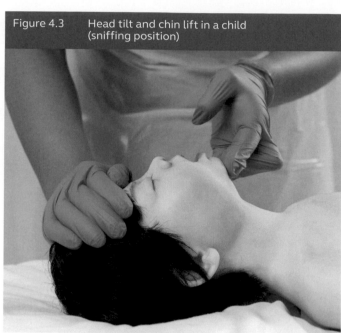

Figure 4.3   Head tilt and chin lift in a child (sniffing position)

S – Shout for assistance

- If there is only one rescuer, they must not leave the child but shout for "help" as they start BLS.

- In cases where there is more than one rescuer, a second rescuer should call the EMS immediately upon recognition of unconsciousness, preferably using the speaker function of a mobile phone and collect and apply an automated external defibrillator (AED) if feasible.

- A lone rescuer with no phone who is dealing with a child who has a witnessed sudden collapse should suspect that this is a primary cardiac arrest. In this situation, a shockable rhythm is likely, and the child may need defibrillation. Seek help immediately if there is no one to go for you.

Information required when requesting EMS (Table 4.1).

Table 4.1 Information required when requesting EMS

National 999 ambulance request
Is the patient breathing normally?
Precise location/address you are calling from?
What number you are calling from?
What is the reason for your call?
How many casualties?

A Airway

In the unconscious child, the tongue is likely to at least partly occlude their airway. This can usually be overcome by using a head tilt and chin lift manoeuvre or, if necessary, by performing a jaw thrust.

Head tilt and chin lift

This is a simple and effective initial manoeuvre. Turn the child on to their back. To perform the head tilt, approach the child from the side, place one hand on their forehead and gently tilt their head back. In infants, the head should be placed in a neutral position (Figure 4.2). For the child, a 'sniffing' position that causes some extension of the head on the neck will be required (Figure 4.3).

The chin lift is performed by placing the fingertips of the rescuer's other hand on the bony part of the child's lower jaw and lifting the chin upwards. Take care not to compress the soft tissues under the child's jaw as this will occlude the airway.

Jaw thrust

This is the preferred airway opening manoeuvre when cervical spine immobilisation is required. To perform a jaw thrust, approach the child from behind and place hands on either side of the child's head. Two or three fingertips of both hands should be placed under both angles of the child's lower jaw. With thumbs resting gently on the child's cheeks, lift the jaw upwards. The rescuer's elbows should rest on the surface that the child is laid on (Figure 4.4).

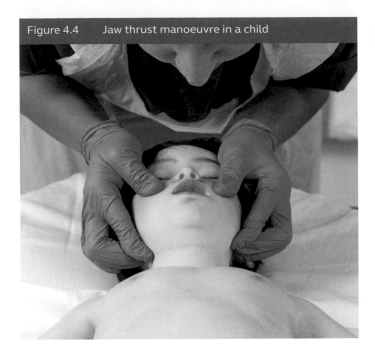

Figure 4.4   Jaw thrust manoeuvre in a child

Have a low threshold for suspecting injury to the neck. If you suspect this, try to open the airway using jaw thrust alone. If this is unsuccessful, add head tilt gradually until the airway is open. Establishing an open airway takes priority over concerns about the cervical spine.

Whichever airway opening method is used, it is also important for rescuers to look in the child's mouth to ensure there is no obvious foreign body present. If a foreign body is seen and the rescuer is confident that they can remove it safely, this can be attempted, but blind finger sweeps should never be performed. The management of choking is discussed later in this chapter.

B Breathing

Assessing for normal breathing

After opening the airway, the rescuer needs to assess the child for effective, normal breathing. The best way to do this is to 'look, listen and feel' whilst maintaining the airway opening manoeuvre.

| LOOK for chest (and abdominal) movements. |

| LISTEN for airflow at the mouth and nose (+/- additional noises). |

| FEEL for airflow at the mouth and nose. |

Keeping the airway open, look, listen, and feel for normal breathing by putting your face close to the child's face and looking along the chest whilst simultaneously looking for signs of life (Figures 4.5 and 4.6).

Signs of life include:

- swallowing
- vocalising
- coughing
- normal (not agonal) breathing.

Look, listen and feel for breath and chest movement

- Listen at the child's nose and mouth for breath sounds.
- Feel for air movement on your cheek.
- In the first few minutes after cardiorespiratory arrest, a child may be taking infrequent, noisy gasps. Do not confuse this with normal breathing.

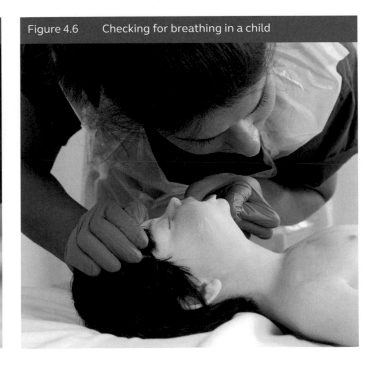

Figure 4.5   Checking for breathing in an infant

Figure 4.6   Checking for breathing in a child

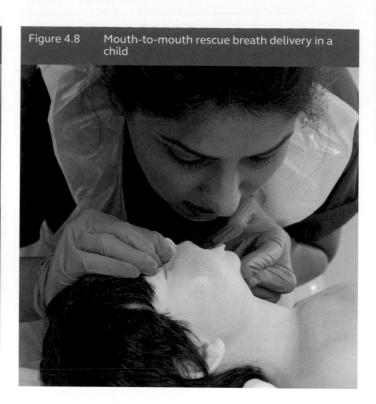

Figure 4.7   Mouth-to-mouth and nose rescue breath delivery in an infant

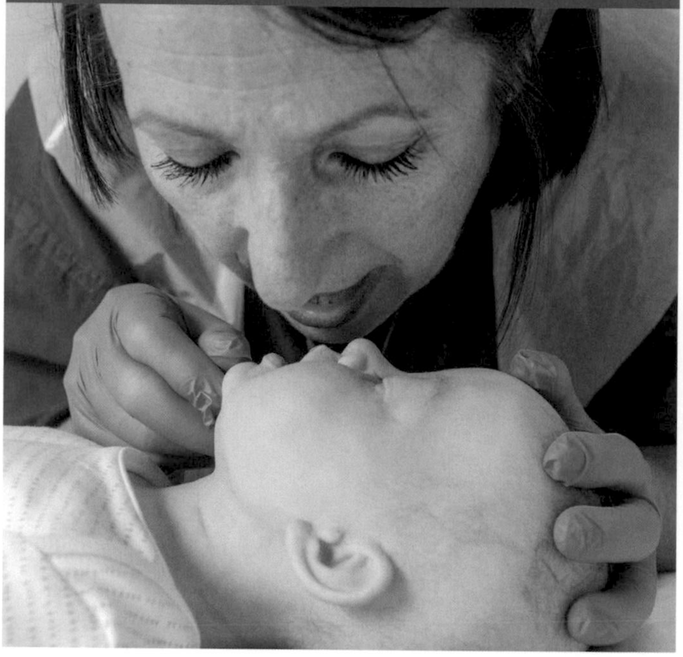

Figure 4.8   Mouth-to-mouth rescue breath delivery in a child

- Look, listen, and feel for no more than 10 s before deciding – if you have any doubts whether breathing is normal, act as if it is not normal.
- Simultaneously look for signs of life.

If the child is breathing normally

- Consider turning the child onto their side into a recovery position (Figure 4.18) or maintain an open airway with a head tilt and chin lift or jaw thrust.
    - If not already done so, call the relevant emergency number (999) on your mobile phone where possible, using the speaker function if available. Only leave the child if no other way of obtaining help is possible.
    - Check for continued normal breathing.

If the child's breathing is NOT normal or absent

- Give 5 initial rescue breaths:
    - While performing the rescue breaths, note any gag or cough response to your action. These responses, or their absence, will form part of your ongoing assessment of signs of life.
    - BLS can be undertaken without any adjuncts; however, expired air ventilation provides only 16–17% of oxygen. Oxygen should be given as soon as possible. The trained healthcare provider must provide bag-mask ventilation (BMV) with oxygen as soon as the necessary equipment is available.

Rescue breaths for an infant (Figure 4.7)
- Ensure a neutral position of the head (as an infant's head is usually flexed when supine, this may require some gentle extension) and apply chin lift.
- Take a breath and cover the mouth and nose of the infant with your mouth, making sure you have a good seal.
- If the nose and mouth cannot both be covered in the older infant, the rescuer may attempt to seal only the infant's nose or mouth with his mouth (if the nose is used, close the lips to prevent air escape).
- Blow steadily into the infant's mouth and nose over 1 s, sufficient to make the chest rise visibly (this is the same time as in adult practice).
- Maintain head position and chin lift, take your mouth away, and watch for the chest to fall as air comes out.
- Take another breath and repeat this sequence four more times.
- Identify effectiveness by seeing the infant's chest rising and falling similarly to the movement produced by a normal breath.

Rescue breaths for a child over 1 year (Figure 4.8)
- Ensure head tilt and chin lift, extending the head into a 'sniffing' position.
- Pinch the soft part of the nose closed with the index finger and thumb of your hand on their forehead.

- Open the mouth a little but maintain a chin lift.
- Take a breath and place your lips around the mouth, making sure you have a good seal.
- Blow steadily into their mouth over 1 s sufficient to make the chest rise visibly.
- Maintain head tilt and chin lift, take your mouth away and watch for the chest to fall as air comes out.
- Take another breath and repeat this sequence four more times.
- Identify effectiveness by seeing the child's chest rising and falling similarly to the movement produced by a normal breath.

For both infants and children, if you have difficulty achieving an effective breath, the airway may be obstructed:

- Open the child's mouth and remove any visible obstruction. Do not perform a blind finger sweep.
- Ensure that there is adequate head tilt and chin lift but also that the neck is not overextended; try repositioning the head to open the airway.
- If head tilt and chin lift has not opened the airway, try the jaw thrust method.
- Take up to 5 attempts to achieve an effective breath. If still unsuccessful, move on to chest compressions.

If there is only one rescuer with a mobile phone, they should call for help (and activate the speaker function) immediately after the 5 initial rescue breaths. Proceed to the next step while waiting for an answer. If no phone is readily available, perform 1 min of CPR before leaving the child. To minimise the interruption in CPR it may be possible to carry an infant or small child whilst summoning help.

In cases where paediatric BLS providers are unable or unwilling to start with ventilations, they should proceed with chest compressions and add ventilations into the sequence as soon as this can be done.

Following the rescue breaths if you are confident that you can detect signs of life:

- Continue rescue breathing (12–30 breaths min^{-1} or as guided by EMS dispatcher) if necessary until the child starts breathing effectively on their own.
- Unconscious children and infants who are not in cardiorespiratory arrest and clearly have normal breathing can have their airway kept open by either continued head tilt and chin lift or jaw thrust or, when there is perceived risk of vomiting, by positioning the unconscious child in a recovery position.
- Reassess the child frequently.

c Circulation

Following the rescue breaths, if there are no signs of life or you are unsure, immediately start high-quality chest compressions.

Principles of chest compressions

Chest compressions are serial, rhythmic compressions of the anterior chest wall, intended to cause blood to flow to vital organ tissues in an attempt to keep them viable until the return of spontaneous circulation (ROSC) is achieved.

High-quality chest compressions

- Rate: 100–120 min^{-1} for both infants and children.
- Depth: depress the lower half of the sternum by at least one-third of the anterior-posterior dimension of the chest (which is approximately 4 cm for an infant and 5 cm for a child).
- Compressions should never be deeper than the adult 6 cm limit (approximately an adult's thumb length).
  - To avoid compressing the upper abdomen, locate the xiphisternum by finding the angle where the lowest ribs join the sternum (breastbone).
  - Compress the sternum one finger's breadth above this.
- Release all pressure on the chest between compressions to allow for complete chest recoil. Avoid leaning on the chest at the end of a compression.
- Allow adequate time for chest recoil to occur (approximately 50% of the whole cycle should be the relaxation phase (i.e. from the start of one compression to the next)).
- After 30 chest compressions, tilt the head, lift the chin, and give 2 rescue breaths.
- Continue compressions and breaths in a ratio of 30:2 (healthcare professionals with a duty to respond to paediatric emergencies may use the ratio of 15:2 as described later in this chapter).
- Perform compressions on a firm surface.
- Pauses in chest compressions should be minimised so that 80% or more of the CPR cycle is comprised of chest compressions.
- The best method for compressions varies slightly between infants and children.

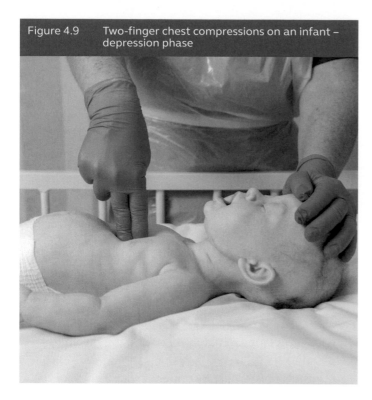

Figure 4.9   Two-finger chest compressions on an infant – depression phase

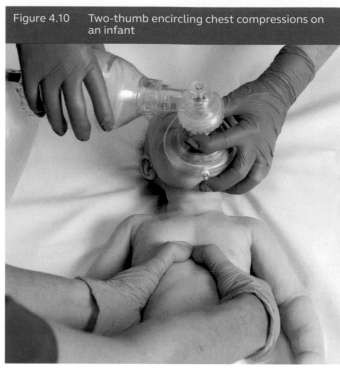

Figure 4.10   Two-thumb encircling chest compressions on an infant

Chest compressions in infants

Two-finger technique

This is the recommended method of infant chest compressions for the lone rescuer. Having landmarked as described above, place two fingers of one hand in the correct position on the sternum and depress it by at least one-third of the depth of the infant's chest, approximately 4 cm (Figure 4.9).

Two-thumb encircling technique

This is the recommended method of infant chest compressions for two rescuers. There is evidence that this method delivers greater cardiac output than the two-finger technique but is difficult for a single rescuer to perform and also deliver timely and effective rescue breaths. It is, therefore, usually reserved for in-hospital resuscitation where there are two rescuers and ventilation delivery devices should be used.

The encircling technique

- Place both thumbs flat, side-by-side, on the lower half of the sternum (as above), with the tips pointing towards the infant's head.
- Spread the rest of both hands, with the fingers together, to encircle the lower part of the infant's ribcage with tips of the fingers supporting the infant's back. Press down on the lower sternum with your two thumbs to depress it at least one-third of the depth of the infant's chest, approximately 4 cm (Figure 4.10).
- For small infants, you may need to overlap your thumbs to provide effective compressions.

Chest compressions in children aged over 1 year

- Place the heel of one hand over the lower half of the sternum (as above).
- Lift the fingers to ensure that pressure is not applied over the child's ribs.
- Position yourself vertically above the child's chest and, with your arm straight, compress the sternum by at least one-third of the depth of the chest, approximately 5 cm (Figure 4.11).
- In larger children, or for small rescuers, this may be achieved by using both hands with fingers interlocked (Figure 4.12).

Do not interrupt CPR at any moment unless there are clear signs of life (normal breathing, coughing, purposeful movement). To prevent fatigue and therefore reduction in the quality of chest compressions delivered, two of more rescuers should alternate who is performing chest compressions. Additionally, the compressing rescuer should alternate the hand which undertakes compressions, or change technique (one to two-handed) to maintain effective compressions.

Continue resuscitation until:

- the child shows signs of life (e.g. normal breathing, coughing, movement)
- additional qualified help arrives
- the rescuer becomes exhausted.

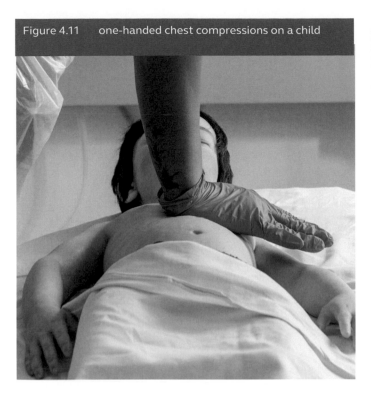

Figure 4.11   one-handed chest compressions on a child

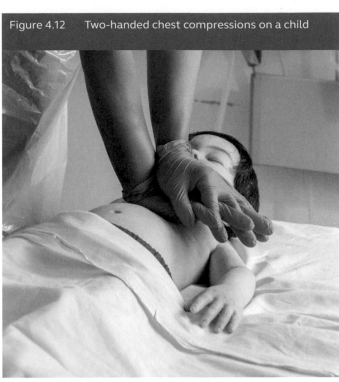

Figure 4.12   Two-handed chest compressions on a child

Automated external defibrillators (AEDs)

- In children and infants with cardiorespiratory arrest, a lone rescuer should immediately start CPR.

- In cases where the likelihood of a primary shockable rhythm is extremely high, such as in sudden witnessed collapse, the lone rescuer should activate the EMS and apply an AED if readily available. When there is more than one rescuer, a second rescuer will immediately call for help and then collect and apply an AED (if available) while the first rescuer continues with CPR.

- Trained providers should limit the no-flow time when using an AED by performing CPR up to the point of analysis and immediately after the shock delivery or no shock decision; pads should be applied with minimal or no interruption in CPR.

- If possible, use an AED with a paediatric attenuator in infants and children below 8 years (energy reduced to 50–75 J). If this is not available, use a standard AED for all ages.

- There have been continuing reports of safe and successful use of AEDs in children less than 8 years, demonstrating that AEDs can identify arrhythmias accurately in children and are extremely unlikely to advise a shock inappropriately.

In-hospital BLS

The following is the sequence to be used by health care professionals with a duty to respond to paediatric emergencies (Figure 4.13).

S	Safety
S	Stimulate
S	Shout for assistance
A	Airway
B	Breathing
C	Circulation

S – Safety

In all emergencies, quickly assess the situation and ensure the safety of first the rescuer(s) and then that of the child; although the potential hazards may be different, this is equally important whether the situation occurs within or outside the healthcare environment.

All bodily fluids should be treated as potentially infectious; put on the required level of personal protective equipment (PPE).

S – Stimulate

Check for a response as described earlier.

If the child responds:

- assess ABCDE (O_2, monitoring, vascular access)
- call for further assistance as appropriate.

S – Shout for assistance

If there is no response:

- call for help/emergency buzzer
- activate 2222 for a clinical emergency team.

Information required when requesting in-hospital clinical emergency team - 2222
Precise location of the emergency
Specific clinical emergency team required (e.g. paediatric resuscitation, paediatric trauma)
Any other local policy requirements

A Airway

Position the child on their back, open and assess the airway as previously described.

B Breathing

Assess for normal breathing whilst simultaneously looking for signs of life. Studies have shown how unreliable feeling for a pulse is in determining the presence or absence of a circulation even for trained paediatric healthcare workers, hence the importance of looking for signs of life. However, if a health care worker still wishes to check for a pulse, this should be done simultaneously with the breathing assessment.

If the child is breathing normally

- Consider turning the child onto their side into a recovery position (Figure 4.18) or maintain an open airway with a head tilt and chin lift or jaw thrust.
  - check for continued normal breathing
  - check ABCDE and treat as required.

If the child's breathing is NOT normal or absent

- Give 5 initial rescue breaths.
  - Provide ventilation initially by bag-mask ventilation (BMV), using high concentration inspired oxygen 100% as soon as possible. To provide an adequate seal of the mask a two-person technique is advocated. (Chapter 3, Figure 3.11)

Following the rescue breath, if you are confident that you can detect signs of life:

- Continue BMV if necessary until the child starts breathing effectively on their own or until the arrival of the in-hospital clinical emergency team.

C Circulation

Following the rescue breaths, if there are no signs of life or if you are unsure, immediately start high-quality chest compressions.

High-quality chest compressions

- Rate: 100–120 min⁻¹ for both infants and children.
- Depth: depress the lower half of the sternum by at least one-third of the anterior-posterior dimension of the chest (which is approximately 4 cm for an infant and 5 cm for a child).
- Compressions should never be deeper than the adult 6 cm limit.
- Release all pressure on the chest between compressions to allow for complete chest recoil and avoid leaning on the chest at the end of a compression.
- Allow adequate time for chest recoil to occur (approximately 50% of the whole cycle should be the relaxation phase (i.e. from the start of one compression to the next)).
- Chest compression pauses should be minimised so that 80% or more of the CPR cycle is comprised of chest compressions.

Chest compressions in infants

Preferably use the two thumb encircling method; if this is not possible, use the two-finger technique.

Chest compressions in children over 1 year

Use one hand; for larger children or smaller rescuers, use both hands with fingers interlocked.

- landmarks for chest compressions are as described earlier in this chapter
- continue chest compressions and breaths at a ratio of 15:2
- attach ECG monitoring/defibrillator when available, minimising any interruptions to CPR.

Continue with this sequence until the arrival of the in-hospital clinical emergency team or until the child starts to show signs of life.

Paediatric basic life support

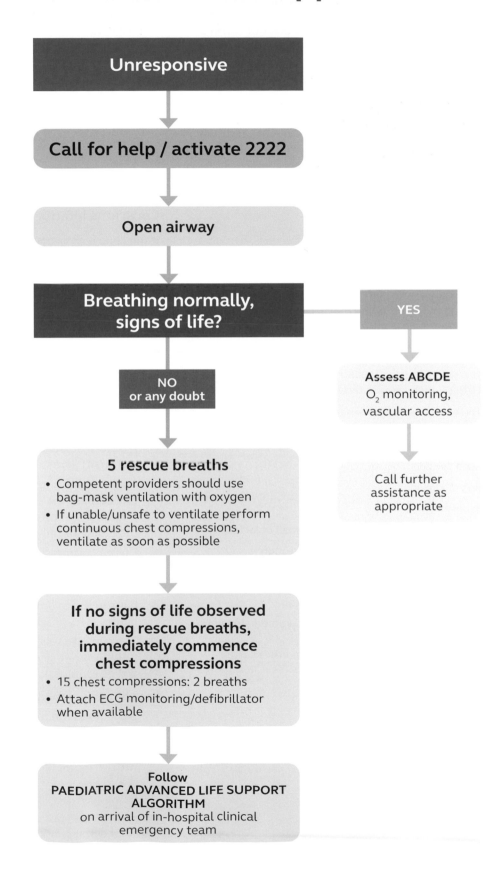

Figure 4.13   Paediatric basic life support algorithm

Choking

When a foreign body enters their airway, a child will react immediately by coughing in an attempt to expel it. A child who is choking on a foreign body but can still cough effectively must be actively encouraged to do so. A spontaneous cough is not only safer, but it is probably more effective than any manoeuvre a rescuer might perform.

However, if coughing is absent or becoming ineffective, the child's airway is at risk of complete obstruction, which will rapidly result in asphyxiation. Any child, who is unable to effectively cough as a result of foreign body aspiration, requires immediate interventions (Figure 4.14).

Recognition of choking

Choking is characterised by the sudden onset of respiratory distress associated with coughing, gagging or stridor.

The majority of choking events in infants and children occur during play or feeding and are frequently witnessed by an adult, which means interventions can start immediately. However, it is important to be aware that the signs of choking (Table 4.2) can be confused with those of other causes of airway obstruction (e.g. laryngitis or epiglottitis), which require different management.

Table 4.2 Signs of choking

General signs	
Witnessed episode	
Coughing or choking	
Sudden onset	
Recent history of playing with or eating small objects	
Ineffective cough	Effective cough
Unable to vocalise	Crying or verbal response to questions
Quiet or silent cough	Loud cough
Unable to breathe	Able to take a breath before coughing
Cyanosis	Fully responsive
Decreasing level of consciousness	

Management of choking

If the child is coughing effectively, no external manoeuvre is necessary. Encourage the child to cough and observe them closely.

If the child's coughing is absent or becoming ineffective, shout for help and quickly determine the child's conscious level.

Management of obstructed airway in-hospital may include the use of suction/laryngoscopy/magills forceps by experienced personnel. Out of hospital, the use of existing anti-choking devices in the first aid of a choking infant/child is not recommended due to the lack of available evidence to date.

Conscious infants and children

If the child is conscious, but their coughing is absent or ineffective, deliver back blows. These are intended to loosen the object for the child to be able to then expel it. If back blows do not relieve the airway obstruction, thrusts should be given; chest thrusts for infants and abdominal thrusts for children. These thrusts are intended as an 'artificial cough'; they increase the intrathoracic pressure, which will facilitate the expulsion of the foreign body.

Back blows in an infant (Figure 4.15)
- Support the infant in a head-downwards, prone position to enable gravity to assist in removing the foreign body.
- A seated or kneeling rescuer should be able to support the infant across his lap.
- Support the infant's head by placing the thumb of one hand at the angle of the lower jaw and one or two fingers from the same hand at the same point on the other side of the jaw.
- Do not compress the soft tissues under the infant's jaw, as this will exacerbate the airway obstruction.
- Deliver up to 5 sharp back blows with the heel of one hand in the middle of the back between the shoulder blades.
- The aim is to relieve the obstruction with each blow rather than to give all 5 (hence, if successful all 5 may not be required).

Back blows in a child over 1 year (Figure 4.16)
- Back blows are more effective if the child is positioned head down.
- A small child may be placed across the rescuer's lap as with an infant. If this is not possible, support the child in a forward-leaning position and deliver the back blows from behind.

If back blows do not relieve the airway obstruction, and the child is still conscious, give chest thrusts to infants or abdominal thrusts to children. Do not use abdominal thrusts (Heimlich manoeuvre) for infants.

Paediatric foreign body airway obstruction

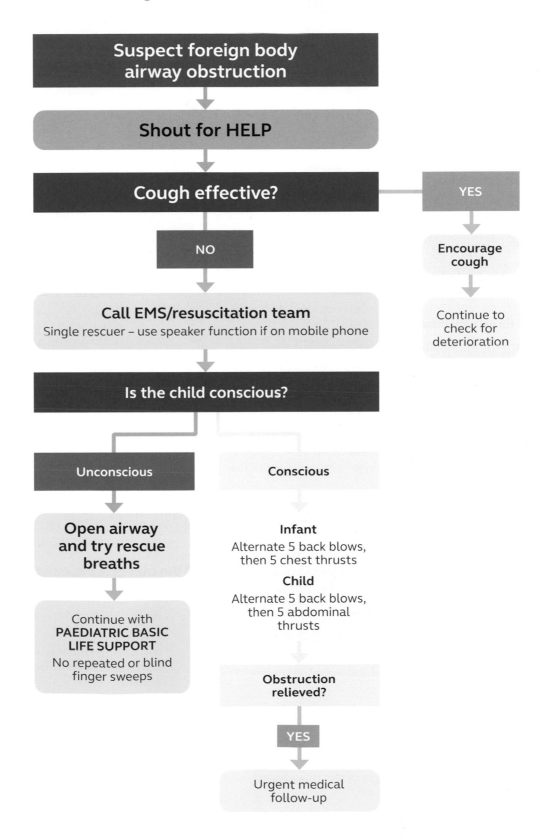

Suspect foreign body airway obstruction

↓

Shout for HELP

↓

Cough effective? ——— **YES**

NO

↓   ↓

Call EMS/resuscitation team
Single rescuer – use speaker function if on mobile phone

Encourage cough

↓   ↓

Is the child conscious?

Continue to check for deterioration

Unconscious   **Conscious**

↓   ↓

Open airway and try rescue breaths

Infant
Alternate 5 back blows, then 5 chest thrusts

Child
Alternate 5 back blows, then 5 abdominal thrusts

↓   ↓

Continue with **PAEDIATRIC BASIC LIFE SUPPORT**
No repeated or blind finger sweeps

Obstruction relieved?

↓

YES

↓

Urgent medical follow-up

Figure 4.14   Paediatric foreign body airway obstruction algorithm

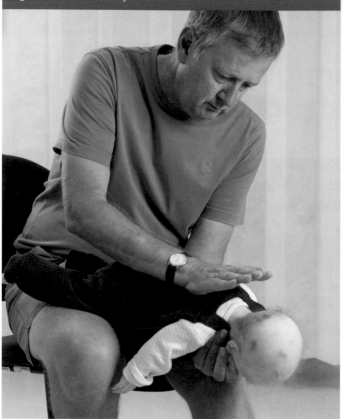

Figure 4.15   Delivery of back blows to an infant

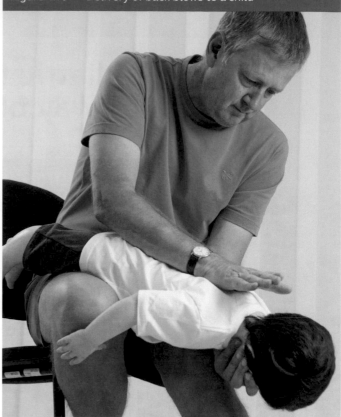

Figure 4.16   Delivery of back blows to a child

Chest thrusts for infants

- Turn the infant into a head-downwards supine position. This is achieved safely by placing your free arm along the infant's back and encircling the occiput with your hand.

- Support the infant down your arm, which is placed down (or across) your thigh.

- Identify the landmark for chest compressions (lower sternum approximately a finger's breadth above the xiphisternum).

- Deliver up to 5 chest thrusts. These are similar to chest compressions but sharper in nature and delivered at a slower rate.

- The aim is to relieve the obstruction with each thrust rather than to give all 5 (hence, if successful all 5 may not be required).

Abdominal thrusts for children over 1 year (Figure 4.17)

- Stand or kneel behind the child. Place your arms under the child's arms and encircle their torso.

- Clench your fist and place it between the umbilicus and xiphisternum.

- Grasp your fist with the other hand and pull sharply inwards and upwards.

- Repeat up to 4 more times.

- Ensure that pressure is not applied to the xiphoid process or the lower rib cage as this may cause abdominal trauma.

- The aim is to relieve the obstruction with each thrust rather than to give all 5 (hence, if successful all 5 may not be required).

Following chest or abdominal thrusts, reassess the infant/child

- If the object has not been expelled and the individual is still conscious, continue the sequence of back blows and chest thrusts for an infant or abdominal thrusts for children.

- Call out, or send for help if it is still not available.

- Do not leave the infant/child at this stage.

- If the object has not been expelled and the infant/child is still conscious, continue the sequence.

If the object is expelled successfully

- Assess the infant or child's clinical condition.

- It is possible that part of the object may remain in the respiratory tract and cause complications.

- If there is any doubt or if the child was treated with abdominal thrusts, urgent medical follow up is mandatory.

If the infant/child with foreign body airway obstruction is, or becomes, unconscious, move to treatment with the paediatric BLS algorithm.

Call for help if it is still not available.

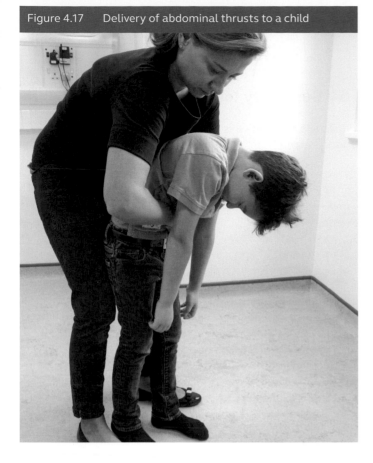

Figure 4.17   Delivery of abdominal thrusts to a child

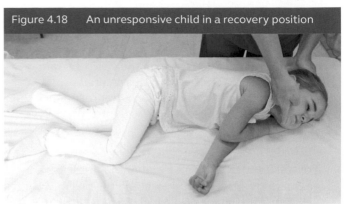

Figure 4.18   An unresponsive child in a recovery position

Airway opening

- When the airway is opened for attempted delivery of rescue breaths, look to see if the foreign body can be seen in the mouth.
- If an object is seen, attempt to remove it with a single finger sweep.
- Do not attempt blind or repeated finger sweeps; these can push the object more deeply into the pharynx and cause injury.

Rescue breaths

- Open the airway and attempt 5 rescue breaths.
- Assess the effectiveness of each breath: if a breath does not make the chest rise, reposition the head before making the next attempt.

Chest compressions and CPR

- Proceed immediately to chest compressions regardless of whether the breaths are successful and perform CPR as previously described.
- Continue with paediatric BLS using a compression and ventilation ratio of 15:2 (or the ratio you are familiar with) until help arrives or the child improves.
- If the child regains consciousness and is breathing effectively, place them in the recovery position and monitor breathing and conscious level whilst awaiting the EMS/in-hospital clinical emergency team.

Recovery position

For children and infants with a decreased level of consciousness who do not meet the criteria for the initiation of rescue breathing or chest compressions (CPR), the recovery position may be recommended (Figure 4.18). The following describes one method of achieving a left lateral position:

- Kneel beside the child and make sure that both their legs are straight.
- Place their arm nearest to you out at a right angle to the body, elbow bent with the hand palm uppermost.
- Bring their far arm across the chest, and hold the back of their hand against the child's cheek nearest to you.
- With your other hand, grasp their far leg just above the knee and pull it up, keeping the foot on the ground.
- Keeping their hand pressed against the cheek, pull on their far leg to roll the child towards you onto their side.
- Adjust their upper leg so that both hip and knee are bent at right angles.
- Tilt the head back to make sure the airway remains open.
- Adjust their hand under the cheek if necessary to keep the head tilted and facing downwards to allow liquid material to drain from the mouth.
- Check breathing regularly.
- Ensure the position is stable. In an infant, this may require the support of a small pillow or a rolled-up blanket placed behind their back to maintain the position.

It is important to maintain a close check on all unconscious individuals until the EMS arrives to ensure that their breathing remains normal (check breathing at least once every minute).

Avoid any pressure on the child or infant's chest that may impair breathing and regularly turn the unconscious child or infant over onto their opposite side to prevent pressure injuries whilst in the recovery position (i.e. every 30 min).

In certain situations, such as when the child or infant is breathing spontaneously but requires airway management, the recovery position is not recommended. In these circumstances:

- Keep the patient flat, maintain an open airway by either continued head tilt and chin lift or jaw thrust
- For a child or infant with traumatic injuries, leave them lying flat, open and maintain their airway using a jaw thrust, taking care to avoid spinal rotation.

04: Summary learning

Rescuers must always ensure their own safety before undertaking BLS.

The preferred ratio of chest compressions : ventilations is 15:2 when BLS is being delivered by healthcare professionals , but in some instances, it may be appropriate to adopt the standard adult 30:2 sequence.

Management of conscious choking infants consists of back blows followed by chest thrusts.

Management of conscious choking children consists of back blows followed by abdominal thrusts.

Management of unconscious infants and children as a result of choking requires BLS to be performed.

My key take-home messages from this chapter are:

Further reading

Kitamura T, Iwami T, Kawamura T, Nagao K, Tanaka H, Nadkarni VM, et al. Conventional and chest-compression-only cardiopulmonary resuscitation by bystanders for children who have out-of-hospital cardiac arrests: a prospective, nationwide, population-based cohort study. Lancet. 2010 Apr 17;375(9723):1347-54.

Kao PC, Chiang WC, Yang CW, Chen SJ, Liu YP, Lee CC, et al. What is the correct depth of chest compression for infants and children? A radiological study. Pediatrics. 2009 Jul;124(1):49-55.

Berg RA, Hilwig RW et al. "Simulated mouth-to-mouth ventilation and chest compressions (bystander cardiopulmonary resuscitation) improves outcome in a swine model of prehospital pediatric asphyxial cardiac arrest." Crit Care Med 1999; 27(9):1893-1899.

Tibballs J, Russell P. Reliability of pulse palpation by healthcare personnel to diagnose paediatric cardiac arrest. Resuscitation. 2009 Jan;80(1):61-4.

Couper K, Hassan A, Ohri V, Patterson E, Tang H, Bingham R, Olasveengen T, Perkins G. On behalf of the International Liaison Committee on Resuscitation Basic and Paediatric Life Support Task Force Collaborators. Removal of foreign body airway obstruction: A systematic review of interventions. Resuscitation 2020; 156:174-181 .

P. Van de Voorde, et al., European Resuscitation Council Guidelines 2021: Paediatric Life Support, Resuscitation (2021), https://doi.org/10.1016/j.resuscitation.2021.02.015.

Pre-hospital care

For the purposes of the chapter, the term 'child' will include neonate and infant.

Team approach and safety in the pre-hospital environment

Assessing and managing children out of the hospital environment brings a different set of challenges. The team is smaller, specialist help is not immediately available, safety is crucial, and the environment can be difficult to operate in.

Safety has been discussed in previous chapters, and this has further emphasis when working in an unfamiliar environment. The emergency services have had training and have experience in working in these situations. They will assess safety by specifically assessing the scene for any hazards, assessing any potential danger to themselves (so that they don't become a further casualty) and assessing the situation of the patient(s). Scene safety could include stopping the traffic before approaching the casualty, and therefore it is recommended to take a short pause beforehand to assess safety.

Environmental factors such as temperature extremes, adverse weather, noise, and movement can affect the child's condition and make a clinical assessment more difficult. Sometimes it will be necessary to move a child to an area where 360° access to the child is possible to allow a more thorough assessment. This could be another room in a house or in the back of an ambulance.

Depending on the number and composition of the team, the team members may not be known to each other prior to arriving at the scene. Bystanders may know the casualty (such as family members), or they may be a trained first aider who was nearby. It is imperative to quickly work out who is present and what skills they have so that that team members can take up the most appropriate roles. Family members can help console an unwell child and give you essential information to help diagnose the problem and present a timeline of events.

The ambulances services in the UK use a publication called JRCALC (Joint Royal Colleges Ambulance Liaison Committee), which standardises the management of patients. This includes an 'age per page' section which, depending on the child's age, gives a weight with corresponding drug doses. If you are first on scene and the child is unresponsive and unknown to bystanders, it may be possible to ascertain the child's approximate age by checking the label on their clothes.

Depending on the situation described to the ambulance call handler, the speed of the ambulance response and composition of the team members will vary. In seriously unwell children and those in cardiorespiratory arrest, an immediate response will be activated. This may occur while the call handler is taking further information or giving life-saving advice over the telephone. Multiple ambulance personnel, including paramedics, will be dispatched. Additionally, a pre-hospital critical care team may be sent to provide specialist skills at the scene (e.g. major trauma, cardiorespiratory arrest) via road or helicopter. These specialist teams, which have doctors with pre-hospital training, are able to supplement the management provided by paramedics (e.g. advanced analgesia, emergency anaesthesia, red cell administration and surgical procedures).

Initial assessment of the unwell or injured child in the pre-hospital environment

In Chapter 2 (Recognition and initial management of the seriously ill child), the ABCDE assessment was discussed. In the pre-hospital setting <C>AcBCDE may be used instead; <C> recognises the need to check for possible catastrophic haemorrhage and Ac takes into account possible cervical spinal injury as part of airway (Table 5.1).

Depending on the situation, during the safety assessment, and before approaching the child, gain any history of what has happened; the trained responder should decide on the best assessment approach. If there is a history of trauma or obvious injuries, the <C>AcBCDE is the most suitable approach. If the child is seriously unwell due to a medical complaint, then the ABCDE is appropriate. If there is any doubt or if both a serious illness and injury are present, then the <C>AcBCDE approach should be used.

Table 5.1   The <C>AcBCDE approach

Treat first what kills first	
<C>	Catastrophic external haemorrhage control
Ac	Airway and cervical spine stabilisation
B	Breathing
C	Circulation
D	Disability neurological status (AVPU, pupils, posture)
E	Exposure (and Environment) – undress the child, keep them warm and understand the history and consequences of the traumatic event

<C> Catastrophic external haemorrhage

If catastrophic external haemorrhage is present, for example, an amputated limb, injured femoral artery or open long bone fracture, this needs to be managed first. This is because the continued bleeding will lead to the child dying of hypovolaemic shock from exsanguination, despite any ABC interventions. Therefore, if large amounts of external bleeding are present, direct pressure with a dressing should be applied.

The ambulance service will carry haemostatic dressings that help the blood clot and further reduce blood loss. Continuously pressing with your fingers will provide more direct pressure than your palm. Releasing the pressure will likely restart the bleeding, and therefore removing the pressure to reassess the injury is not advised.

Haemorrhage from a limb is managed with a tourniquet being applied to a long bone above the injury. These can be improvised using a belt or scarf by wrapping it around the limb once and then twisting the ends until it tightens. Clinically designed tourniquets are carried by the emergency ambulance crews and may be used if they are immediately available. If the child is conscious, the amount of compression caused by the tourniquet will likely be painful; strong analgesia will be required.

The child should be transported to hospital as a priority, and if a tourniquet is applied, the time it was first applied must be passed on to the ambulance service ready to handover to the hospital trauma team.

Ac Airway with in-line cervical spine immobilisation

The airway should be managed as discussed in previous chapters, and a stepwise approach may be required if the clinical situation is dynamically changing.

If there is potential for a cervical spinal injury, cervical immobilisation management will also need to be performed. Additionally, if there is concern about a spinal injury, the jaw thrust technique should be used and not a head tilt chin lift.

When assessing the airway outside, it may be more difficult to hear breath sounds with or without a stethoscope. You may need to reassess this again when the child has been moved to somewhere quieter. Looking and feeling may need to be relied upon more than usual initially.

B Breathing

Assessment of breathing should be performed as you would usually do during an ABCDE assessment. As above, if the ambient noise is loud, certain aspects of the examination may not be successfully performed. They can be done once the noise has dissipated. If the child is cold, the saturation probe may not be accurate, and it may also be affected by movement artefact in a moving ambulance.

In critically ill children, those presenting with acute hypoxaemia or in the peri-arrest situation give high-concentration oxygen immediately via a non-rebreathe mask with reservoir.

For children who demonstrate absent or inadequate breathing, assisted ventilation may be required. BMV with or without airway adjuncts is the simplest and safest method of providing this in children. Use of advanced airways (SGA, TT) should only be inserted by those experienced in their use and if BMV is ineffective. Whilst tracheal intubation provides a definitive airway, it is more challenging in the pre-hospital environment, and it can be more difficult to detect complications (e.g. prolonged desaturation, unrecognised oesophageal intubation, bronchial intubation); additionally, for most children, there have been no demonstrated advantages of early intubation. If an advanced airway is used, capnography should be used to confirm the airway's placement and monitor for complications.

C Circulation

The assessment of circulation should follow the same process as described earlier. It may not be possible to measure a non-invasive blood pressure, depending on the availability of appropriately sized blood pressure cuffs. Establishing vascular access may be more difficult compared to a healthcare environment. The positioning of the child, expertise in cannulating infants, acute stress/pain and a cold environment can add to an already challenging situation. In some circumstances, intraosseous access will be required in seriously unwell children.

D Disability

Frequently assess and reassess AVPU. This is a good marker of improvement or deterioration in a seriously unwell child. The pupillary response, posture and tone of the child should be assessed. Glucose can easily be measured and is often low in an unwell child. Oral glucose or IM glucagon can be administered if IV is difficult. Glucagon is used to release glucose into the bloodstream from the body's glycogen stores. Paramedics can administer it to children who have a reduced conscious level due to hypoglycaemia when IV access is difficult.

E Exposure

Examination of other areas needs to be weighed against exposure to the cold, wind or rain. The child's and family's privacy needs need to be respected too. So, if possible, exposure should be limited and brief if required. Otherwise, it should be completed once in a warm and sheltered environment, such as indoors or in an ambulance.

Drowning

Drowning causes respiratory impairment from immersion (at least face and upper airway covered) or submersion (all the body) in water or another fluid. The most common and detrimental consequence of drowning is hypoxia. The duration of hypoxia is the critical factor in determining the outcome.

Terms such as dry or wet drowning, near-drowning or silent drowning should not be used.

S – Safety

Personal safety is always a priority. Attempt to save the child without entry into the water. Try to reach the child with a rescue aid (e.g. stick, clothing), throwing a rope or a buoyant rescue aid or using a boat. If entry into the water is essential, a floating device (e.g. buoyant rescue aid) should be used.

The child should be removed from the water by the fastest and safest means available. Remove the individual from the water in a horizontal position (if possible) to avoid post-drowning hypotension and cardiovascular collapse.

A Airway

Cervical spine injury is rare, and c-spine immobilisation is difficult to perform in the water. Therefore, c-spine immobilisation is not indicated unless a severe injury is likely (e.g. diving, waterslide use). Open the airway by jaw thrust if possible.

B Breathing

In-water rescue breathing should be performed only if the rescuer is trained to do so. Otherwise, rescue breathing must be started when out of the water (or in shallow water) if there is no spontaneous breathing after opening the airway.

C Circulation

Assess circulation for hypovolaemic shock and give a bolus of fluid as indicated but avoid fluid overload. If there are no signs of life or a central pulse, start chest compressions.

Hypothermia

Hypothermia is diagnosed when the body's core temperature falls below 35°C; a higher threshold may be considered in infants. Young children are at risk because they have a high body surface area to weight ratio, resulting in a faster rate of heat loss. It is usually a consequence of environmental causes such as drowning and exposure (worse when both wet and windy). However, in teenagers, consider drug and alcohol ingestion as complicating factors; note that sepsis can present with mild hypothermia.

The body regulates falling core temperature by generating heat (e.g. shivering) and by heat conservation (e.g. peripheral vasoconstriction). Early signs and symptoms in children will be cold extremities and shivering (NB infants less than 6 months old do not shiver).

Core temperature is best measured using an oesophageal or rectal thermometer where possible, as tympanic thermometer measurements may be unreliable. Low reading thermometers may be needed in hypothermia.

Hypothermia can be mild, moderate, or severe. The risk of death increases as the core temperature drops below 32°C and temperatures below 28°C are immediately life-threatening (Table 5.2).

Assessment

ABCDE approach, unless suspicion of traumatic injury where an <C>AcBCDE approach may be more appropriate.

- Airway: ensure open and safe.
- Breathing: assess ventilation rate, chest movement and monitor SpO_2 if able to obtain saturation trace.
- Circulation: assess heart rate, rhythm, pulses and monitor blood pressure and ECG for moderate and severe cases.
- Disability: assess level of consciousness, posture, responsiveness, pupil response and blood glucose.
- Environment: accurate assessment of core temperature is very important.

Management

Conscious individuals with mild hypothermia (temperature > 32°C) are usually successfully treated with simple external rewarming measures: remove wet clothes, dry patient, warm blankets, cover with a 'space blanket' and transfer to a warm environment. For infants and small children, cover the head with a hat where possible as the surface area of the head is a large proportion of overall body surface areas. Warm 41°C packs may be used over the chest, abdomen and groins.

Table 5.2   Classification, signs and symptoms of hypothermia

Classification	Temperature	Signs and symptoms	
Mild hypothermia	32–35°C	34–35°C	Shivering +++; pale, cold to touch, quiet and sleepy
		< 34°C	Increasing confusion, altered judgement, fatigue, nausea
		32–33°C	Shivering stops, apathy, ataxia, usually stable haemodynamically but may have atrial arrhythmias
		Tachycardia, tachypnoea, cold diuresis (as kidney loses concentrating ability) – may present as incontinence; may develop red, cold skin and/or hypoglycaemia	
Moderate hypothermia	28–32°C	Bradycardia, hypotension, hypoventilation, hyporeflexia, further reduction LOC	
		Slurred speech, inability to complete simple tasks	
		Atrial arrhythmias	
		28–30°C	Pupils dilated and minimally responsive to light
		28°C	Ventricular arrhythmias (including VF), fixed dilated pupils
Severe hypothermia	< 28°C	Unconscious, unresponsive, fixed pupils, rigid muscles, areflexia, slow shallow breathing (may be just 1 breath per min) or apnoeic	
		VF and further myocardial depression – pulses hard to detect	
		'appears dead'	
		20°C	Asystole

For children with a core temperature below 32°C

- Children with moderate and severe hypothermia should be transferred to hospital for active rewarming.

- Remove wet clothing and cover with dry warm coverings; careful handling is required to prevent precipitating arrhythmias.

- Monitor core temperature, HR and rhythm, check glucose (and electrolytes if possible).

- An echocardiogram may be helpful in the assessment of hypothermic patients when signs of life are absent, pulses are difficult to detect, and the ECG is very slow.

- Open airway, give warmed and humified oxygen.
  - If not breathing, ventilate with high-concentrations of warm, humidified oxygen. The chest wall can be stiff in hypothermia due to muscle rigidity which can make ventilation more difficult.
  - Intubation and other interventions may precipitate VF, so this should be done with care by experts.

- If the child is pulseless, start BLS and assess the heart rhythm; muscle rigidity will make chest compressions more difficult to perform.
  - Hypothermia substantially reduces the effectiveness of defibrillation and resuscitation drugs. It is reasonable to attempt defibrillation, but if this is unsuccessful, continue chest compressions until core temperature > 30°C, when drugs and defibrillation are more likely to be effective. Only give drugs when the core temperature is > 30°C as earlier administration may result in accumulation whilst cold with resultant toxicity when rewarmed. Once 30°C core temperature is reached, give drugs but double the drug dose intervals until 35°C.
  - Never diagnose death and stop cardiopulmonary resuscitation until the patient has been rewarmed to at least 32°C or cannot be rewarmed despite active measures. In some cases, hypothermia can exert a protective effect on the brain, and vital organs and intact neurological recovery can occur even after prolonged cardiorespiratory arrest if deep hypothermia develops before asphyxia.

- Rewarming
  - For patients with altered consciousness, both active external and internal rewarming is required.
  - Active rewarming is best performed in hospital. Methods employed include:
    - Warmed IV fluids: start with pre-warmed 0.9% sodium chloride at 40°C if there is no evidence of hypoglycaemia. Hypokalaemia is common, and electrolytes should be regularly monitored. Patients may require large volumes of fluid during rewarming as vasodilation causes expansion of the intravascular space. Continuous haemodynamic monitoring essential.
    - Gastric or bladder lavage using 0.9% sodium chloride warmed to 40°C.
    - Ventilation with humified gas heated to 42°C.
    - Active external rewarming: overhead warmers and/or warm air system (e.g. Bair hugger, thermal mattress).
  - Check blood gases, potassium, glucose and blood haematocrit with every few degrees of warming.
  - Actively rewarm to 32°C, then allow passive rewarming. Once the patient's core temperature is above the fibrillation threshold of 32°C, there is less urgency in rewarming.
  - Monitor the heart rhythm being aware that peripheral rewarming and vasodilatation can result in cold, acidotic blood being shunted to the core with a drop in temperature, hypotension and again, an increased risk of arrhythmias.
  - Avoid subsequent hyperthermia; keep < 36.5°C.

Pre-hospital management of paediatric illnesses

Once any life-threatening conditions have been identified and managed, more information can be gathered by paramedics or other pre-hospital clinicians. If a child requires an immediate transfer to hospital for further management, this additional information gathering may need to be curtailed or even omitted.

However, if able, a detailed history should be taken from any caregivers present, including the presenting complaint, social and family history, past medical history, previous hospital admissions or recent contact with primary care clinicians. In addition, the history of the child's oral/feeding intake, activity levels, wet nappies, sleeping patterns, immunisation, developmental milestones and any complications during pregnancy or delivery can help formulate a diagnosis. Clues from the environment and interaction with caregivers will also provide valuable information.

The ABCDE assessment approach and treatment of specific illnesses are managed similarly by critical care practitioners to those in hospital guidelines. Some treatments are not available out of hospital (unless an advanced practice paramedic or pre-hospital critical care team are in attendance), and these are listed in Table 5.3. Therefore, the initial treatment of acute illness will be delivered before and during a transfer to hospital. It is often difficult to know if a compensated state will lead to decompensation, especially in children with complex needs or in the very young, and therefore there is a low threshold for further assessment in hospital. Remember that a tiring or exhausted child is an ominous sign, as is a decreasing level of consciousness or responsiveness towards the caregiver.

Table 5.3   Treatments unavailable pre-hospital

Paediatric illness	Treatments unavailable pre-hospital*
Asthma	Intravenous medications – magnesium infusion, aminophylline infusion, salbutamol infusion
Sepsis	Vasoactive infusions (inotropes or vasopressors)
Status epilepticus	3rd line treatment – rapid sequence induction
Hypoglycaemia	Continuous glucose infusion
Ingestion of toxins	Specific antidotes (naloxone available)
*Unless a pre-hospital critical care team is in attendance. Some of these treatments may then be available.	

Out-of-hospital cardiorespiratory arrest in infants and children

Outcomes for children after out-of-hospital (OHCA) are poor. Data on cardiorespiratory arrest in children under 18 years of age from an out-of-hospital cardiac arrest (OHCA) audit in England between January 2014 and December 2018 indicated that there were on average 570 paediatric OHCA per year, with an incidence of cardiorespiratory arrest of 5 per 100 000 children under 18 years of age. The median age of the children was 3.3 years old, and 58% were male. A bystander, family member or EMS crew witnessed the OHCA in one-third of cases; however, only 60% received bystander CPR. A medical cause for OHCA was given for two-thirds of patients, with 7% asphyxiation, 6% trauma, 2% drowning and 1% toxic ingestion The presenting cardiac rhythm was asystole in 66%, with only 6% in a shockable rhythm; an AED was used in just 1.2% of cases.

Overall outcome for ROSC at hospital handover by emergency medical services teams was 18% and survival to hospital discharge of 9%.

Survival after OHCA relies on early recognition and CPR from bystanders. When an ambulance is called, ambulance service telephone dispatchers will assist bystanders in identifying cardiorespiratory arrest and starting CPR before the ambulance arrives. Most paediatric cardiorespiratory arrests are not caused by primary cardiac problems but are secondary to other causes, usually hypoxia. However, in cases where the likelihood of a primary shockable rhythm is extremely high, such as in sudden witnessed collapse, if easily accessible, the bystander/rescuer should apply an automated external defibrillator (AED) at the time of calling EMS. When there is more than one bystander/rescuer, a second bystander/rescuer should immediately call for help and then collect and apply an AED (if feasible).

AEDs are available in many public places (e.g. train stations, shopping centres), and in many areas, the ambulance dispatcher will be able to tell bystanders the location of the nearest AED. There have been continuing reports of safe and successful use of AEDs in children less than 8 years, demonstrating that AEDs can identify arrhythmias accurately in children and are extremely unlikely to advise a shock inappropriately.

A bystander being willing and able to perform timely BLS before the ambulance arrives is crucial in improving outcomes for both children and adults who have an OHCA. This highlights the importance of the Restart a Heart initiative and the inclusion of CPR within the national school curriculums; both initiatives aim to improve the knowledge and skills of a larger number of laypeople who can then deliver bystander CPR. Early BLS, rapid activation of the Emergency Medical Service and prompt, effective advanced life support is crucial in improving mortality and morbidity. Once cardiorespiratory arrest has been confirmed, the sequence of actions in paediatric BLS will depend upon the level of training of the rescuer attending (Chapter 4). These are summarised in Table 5.4.

It is possible for the different ratios of CPR to be delivered to a child in cardiorespiratory arrest. It may mean that as the training of responder increases, there may be a change in compressions: breaths ratio during the early stages of cardiopulmonary resuscitation. The paramedics will then add advanced resuscitation management to the ongoing BLS.

BLS is more effective when the rescuer is proficient in its delivery, but even suboptimal CPR gives a better result than no CPR at all. Hence rescuers unable or unwilling to provide mouth-to-mouth ventilation should be encouraged to perform at least compression-only CPR. A child or infant is far more likely to be harmed if the bystander does nothing.

Debriefing

Following an out-of-hospital resuscitation attempt, an immediate debrief with the attending EMS team can provide both a learning opportunity and support for the team. Debriefing in a structured manner allows a review of the non-technical elements of resuscitation such as communication, leadership and team working. Ideally, the debrief is led by a person trained and capable of leading the session in a constructive manner.

If a defibrillator with the capability to monitor CPR quality has been used, this data can be used to inform the debrief and drive quality improvements.

Out-of-hospital cardiac arrest outcomes (OHCAO) database

Ongoing, systematic collection and analysis of data about out-of-hospital cardiorespiratory arrest and bystander CPR is essential to the planning, implementation, and evaluation of effective CPR programs. The British Heart Foundation and Resuscitation Council UK established a national OHCAO registry in partnership with the National Association of Ambulance Medical Directors and the University of Warwick. The OHCAO registry collects process and outcome information about patients treated by ambulance services for cardiorespiratory arrest and is based on the international Utstein template. The registry will provide a tool to support local quality improvement initiatives and will facilitate measuring the impact of cardiopulmonary resuscitation interventions.

Table 5.4   Type of responder/level of training

Type of responder/level of training	BLS sequence for cardiorespiratory arrest	
Bystander with no CPR training	EMS dispatcher directed CPR – Adult sequence with paediatric modifications	– 5 rescue breaths – 30 chest compressions : 2 breaths
	Chest compressions only	Chest compressions only No mouth-to-mouth breaths
Healthcare provider and lay rescuers trained in 'adult' BLS e.g. first aider or adult based healthcare worker in the vicinity	BLS with paediatric modifications	– 5 rescue breaths – 30 chest compressions : 2 breaths
Healthcare professionals with a duty to respond to paediatric emergencies e.g. paramedic	Paediatric BLS	– 5 initial rescue breaths – 15 chest compressions : 2 breaths

Recognition of life extinct

The pre-hospital care teams will follow protocols when life extinct is ultimately recognised and discuss with local organisations for transfer to hospital for post-bereavement care.

Packaging a patient prior to transfer

The paramedic team will package the patient appropriately depending on the child's condition and/or injuries. This will include lying on the transfer trolley with its standard straps, modified paediatric straps or on a caregiver's lap with a restraint. Injured children may be transferred on a scoop stretcher if it is a short transfer time or in a vacuum mattress. The latter provides immobilisation and insulation.

Pre-alert and patient handover

The receiving emergency department should be alerted as soon as possible if a child is seriously unwell or in cardiorespiratory arrest. A structured method is used by the ambulance services to pass the important pieces of information in a short amount of time. Typically, this is done using 'ATMIST' (Table 5.5) along with an estimated time of arrival and if a specific hospital response is required (for example a resuscitation team or trauma team).

Table 5.5   A structured approach to providing key information – the ATMIST mnemonic

	Medical	Trauma
A	Age	Age
T	Time of onset	Time of incident
M	Medical complaint/history	Mechanism of injury
I	Investigations (brief examination of findings)	Injuries (top to toe)
S	Vital Signs (first set and significant changes)	Vital Signs (first set and significant changes)
T	Treatment, including ETA and any specialist resources needed on arrival	Treatment, including ETA and any specialist resources needed on arrival
ETA – expected time of arrival		

When the pre-hospital team arrive at hospital with the patient, an ATMIST handover is given to the receiving team. Unless CPR is ongoing, this is a hands-off handover so that all the team members can listen to the important information without distraction. Once the handover has been taken, the team leader will then lead the team in the assessment/management of the child.

5: Summary learning

Team approach and safety in the pre-hospital environment.

Initial assessment of the unwell or injured child in the pre-hospital environment.

Drowning children must be removed from water by the fastest and safest means.

Pre-hospital management of paediatric illnesses and cardiopulmonary resuscitation.

Out-of-hospital cardiorespiratory arrest.

Patient packaging, pre-alert and patient handover.

My key take-home messages from this chapter are:

Further reading

Association of Ambulance Chief Executives (Great Britain) & Joint Royal Colleges Ambulance Liaison Committee 2019, JRCALC clinical guidelines 2019, Class Professional Publishing, Bridgwater.

The Out of Hospital Cardiac Arrest Outcome registry warwick ac.uk/fac/sci/med/research/ctu/trials/ohcao

In this chapter

Intravenous access in children during resuscitation

Intraosseous access, advantages and disadvantages

Fluid administration in resuscitation

First-line resuscitation drugs

The learning outcomes will enable you to:

Understand the requirement for circulatory access

Describe the advantages and potential complications of intraosseous access

Understand the type and volume of fluids to be administered in the emergency situation

Know the indications, dosages and actions of the first-line medications used in cardiorespiratory arrest

Circulatory access

Once the airway is patent and adequate ventilation of the child is established, attention must be focused on circulation.

Establish circulatory access within the first few minutes of resuscitation in order that:

- medications (e.g. adrenaline) can be given
- fluids can be started
- blood samples can be obtained.

Circulatory access may be achieved via the intravenous (IV) or intraosseous (IO) routes. In cardiorespiratory arrest and/or severe shock states, when peripheral circulation is severely compromised, the IO route is the preferred method of gaining vascular access. The tracheal route is no longer recommended because of the variability in alveolar drug absorption.

For children who are unwell but remain responsive to pain, IV access is preferred over IO if possible, as infusions of fluids and drugs via the IO route can be painful. If an IV cannula is already in situ, check its patency before use; otherwise, insert the largest possible IV cannula in peripheral veins (e.g. the antecubital fossa, the long saphenous vein or the back of the hand (or feet in smaller children)).

The use of the scalp veins during resuscitation is not advisable owing to the risk of extravasation, leading to potential tissue necrosis. Their use may also interfere with the management of the airway and ventilation. If the child requires chest compressions, these should not be interrupted by access attempts or other procedures apart from defibrillation.

Circulatory access may be achieved via the intravenous (IV) or intraosseous (IO) routes

Intraosseous access

In cardiorespiratory arrest, the IO route is the emergency circulatory access route of choice. Placement of an IO cannula involves inserting a needle through the skin, periosteum and cortex of a bone into the medullary cavity.

The IO route should be the first choice in any situation where the child's clinical status is severely compromised (i.e. they are in a decompensated state) or they have suffered a cardiorespiratory arrest.

The main advantages of IO access are:

- The relative ease and speed of insertion.
- It can be used to deliver all resuscitation fluids, medications and blood-derived products.
- It allows rapid adequate plasma concentration of medications similar to that of central venous administration (more rapid and reliable than that achieved through a peripheral IV).
- It permits bone marrow aspiration, which can be used for analysis. In this situation, the laboratory should be informed as the fat in a marrow sample may cause damage to auto-analysers. There is no point-of-care machine available that is currently licensed to analyse bone marrow.

Insertion of an intraosseous cannula

Before undertaking this procedure, the appropriate equipment must be available, and there should be no contraindications to IO insertion.

Insertion site – anatomical landmarks

The usual site for insertion of an IO cannula is 2–3 cm below the tuberosity on the anteromedial surface of the tibia (Figure 6.1). Other sites that can be used include the lower end of the tibia (approximately 1–3 cm above the medial malleolus) or on the centro-medial aspect of the distal femur (1–2 cm above the patella and 1–2 cm medial to the midline). These sites specifically avoid the growth plates of the bones.

Contraindications
Contraindications to the insertion of an IO include osteogenesis imperfecta ('brittle bone' disease) and haemophilia or other known coagulopathies.
IO cannulation should not be through an area of infected skin or wounds. Fractured bones must not be used, nor should the cannula be inserted into a bone immediately distal to a fracture site, as this may predispose to the development of compartment syndrome.

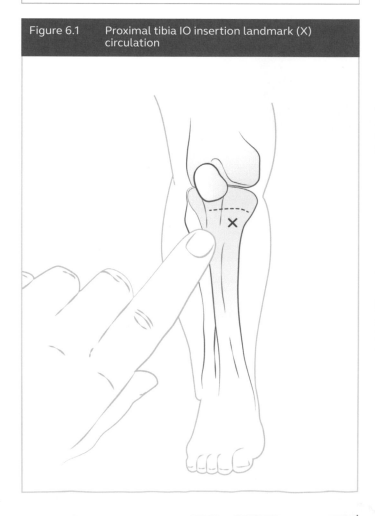

Figure 6.1   Proximal tibia IO insertion landmark (X) circulation

Equipment required

1. IO cannulae

Manual IO cannulae: there are several designs of manually inserted IO cannulae available commercially. They come in a variety of sizes. Generally, it is recommended that size 18 gauge is used for a newborn–6 months of age, 16 gauge for a child between 6–18 months, and 14 gauge for children > 18 months.

Powered IO needle devices: these devices are becoming more popular. One such device is the EZ-IO device which requires minimal practice and training, and results show it to be a safe and rapid means of obtaining IO access. The powered EZ-IO device needles are all 15 gauge but come in a variety of lengths for different weights (15, 25, 45 mm). There is a black 5 mm depth marking on the side of the needle, which should remain visible after pushing the needle through the soft tissue to rest on the periosteum (prior to utilising the drill mechanism); otherwise, the needle will not be long enough to reach the medullary space.

2. Alcohol-based skin preparation solution to minimise the risk of infection.

3. Three-way tap with integrated IV extension tubing primed with 0.9% sodium chloride and attached to a syringe to allow for flushing of medications.

4. Syringe to aspirate bone marrow once the IO is in place (this is not always achievable but will confirm correct position if possible).

5. Emergency medications and/or fluids.

6. Local anaesthetic agent.

If the child is still conscious, this should be considered to minimise pain along the intended track of the IO cannula. Local anaesthetic may also be required once the IO is in place prior to giving fluid and medications, as infusion may be painful via this route.

Potential complications

Although these are uncommon, complications can occur. These include:

- Extravasation: true extravasation ('tissuing') of an IO cannula is uncommon. However, transient swelling of subcutaneous tissue is commonly seen as fluid leaks from the marrow cavity into surrounding tissues. If the swelling does not rapidly subside or there is concern that the cannula is misplaced, the rescuer should withdraw a small amount of fluid; this aspirate should be blood-stained if the cannula is in the correct place.

- Embolism: There is a small risk (estimated at < 1%) of fat or bone marrow embolism.

- Infection: (e.g. osteomyelitis or cellulitis).

- Compartment syndrome: which may result from a large extravasation into a fascial compartment or misplacement of the IO needle. This can compromise the blood supply distally, causing limb ischaemia. This is a more common complication and requires ongoing surveillance and urgent plastic surgery referral if it occurs.

- Skin necrosis.

- Fracture.

The potential for any of the listed complications other than fracture can be minimised by removing the cannula as soon as alternative secure intravenous access has been obtained. Usually, IO needles are removed as soon as another means of vascular access (either peripheral or central) is available and ideally within 24 h.

Fluid administration for volume resuscitation

Intravascular fluids are primarily administered to restore circulatory volume and ensure adequate perfusion of vital organs.

During cardiorespiratory arrest, hypovolaemia is often a primary contributory factor, and fluid resuscitation may play a critical part in achieving the return of spontaneous circulation.

The administration of fluids is also indicated for any child exhibiting signs of circulatory failure (e.g. decreased skin perfusion, prolonged capillary refill time, hypotension). The only children in whom caution is advised are those in suspected cardiogenic shock where the heart is unable to deal with the volume load or those with diabetic ketoacidosis.

Fluid volumes

During the resuscitation of a child with compromised circulation due to hypovolaemia (including sepsis and anaphylaxis), initial resuscitation fluid is administered as a bolus of 10 mL kg^{-1}. The child's circulatory status should then be reassessed, and if signs of circulatory failure persist, this should be repeated. Signs of over-transfusion are moist sounds ('crackles') at the lung bases and jugular venous distension in children or liver distension in infants.

If circulatory failure is due to other causes, such as cardiac failure, a smaller initial volume (5–10 mL kg^{-1}) should be used. The effect of each smaller bolus should be carefully assessed to ensure that fluid administration is not causing worsening of the circulation (e.g. crackles at the lung bases and size of liver edge). The fluid bolus size in trauma is also 10 mL kg^{-1}, followed by careful clinical reassessment because excessive fluid administration in trauma is associated with increased morbidity.

Fluids are indicated during cardiorespiratory arrest if hypovolaemic shock is a likely cause of the arrest. However, excessive amounts should be avoided as fluid overload is counterproductive and may be harmful in post-resuscitation states.

The aim in the management of hypovolaemic shock is to prevent the onset of decompensated circulatory failure, as this may lead to irreversible cardiorespiratory failure and death. Measurement of blood pressure is of little help in determining circulatory status as it remains normal in compensated circulatory failure and only starts to drop as decompensation develops. The principles of management adhere to ABCDE (airway, breathing, circulation, disability, exposure) with fluid administration forming part of the 'C' phase of resuscitation.

Types of fluid

In the initial phase of resuscitation, isotonic salt solutions should be used. There are no clear advantages between using crystalloid or colloid solutions. Glucose-containing solutions (such as dextrose saline) should never be used for volume replacement as they can cause hyponatraemia and hyperglycaemia, which in turn can lead to further fluid loss.

Crystalloids

There may be advantages to using balanced isotonic crystalloid solutions; however, 0.9% sodium chloride is an acceptable and widely available alternative. Examples of balanced crystalloids include Ringer's lactate, Hartmann's solution and Plasma-Lyte or Normosol.

Crystalloids are cheap, readily available and do not cause allergic reactions. Previously they have been considered less effective than colloids at expanding the circulating volume (due to rapid dispersal to the interstitial space), but in practice, this effect is minimal.

Infusion of fluids containing potassium must be used with caution in children with anuria or oliguria, as hyperkalaemia could arise.

Glucose solutions should never be used for volume expansion as they can cause hyperglycaemia, resulting in osmotic diuresis. This increases urine production, and so increases circulatory volume loss. Glucose solutions should only be used to correct hypoglycaemia following measurement of blood sugar levels: 2 mL kg^{-1} of 10% glucose is given, and the patient's blood sugar should be re-measured shortly afterwards to ensure it is within the normal range. In the newborn, 2.5 mL kg^{-1} of 10% glucose may be given initially to correct hypoglycaemia.

Colloids

Examples of colloids include:

- human albumin (4.5%) solution
- fresh frozen plasma (FFP)
- blood.

Colloids are relatively expensive and less readily available than crystalloids; however, in certain circumstances, they may be indicated, for example, to correct coagulopathy in sepsis. Colloids should be not be used in anaphylaxis because of the potential risk of an allergic reaction.

Blood products

The administration of blood products is reserved for situations where there is a specific indication for their use (i.e. blood loss or coagulopathy).

If the infusion of 20 mL kg^{-1} (i.e. 10 mL kg^{-1} bolus x 2) does not improve the circulatory status of a child who has suffered trauma, transfusion of blood must be considered, as well as urgent surgical referral.

In an emergency, Group O Rhesus-negative 'flying squad' blood or type specific uncross-matched blood may be used for transfusion until fully cross-matched blood is available.

The risks of blood product administration must always be borne in mind.

First-line resuscitation medications

Only a few medications are indicated during the initial resuscitation phase of a child in cardiorespiratory arrest. Administration of medications should be considered only after adequate ventilation and chest compressions have been established, and in the case of a shockable arrhythmia (VF or pVT), following delivery of the first three defibrillation shocks.

For safety reasons, as well as speed and ease of use, the use of pre-filled medication syringes is advocated.

All medications administered should be followed by a flush of 2–5 mL 0.9% sodium chloride to ensure they reach the circulation and to minimise the risks of interactions with any other medications or fluids administered via the same cannula. All medications and fluids should be recorded as they are administered and then documented at the end of the resuscitation attempt.

Adrenaline

Indications for use
- cardiorespiratory arrest of any aetiology
- bradycardia < 60 min^{-1} with signs of inadequate perfusion after the initial steps to restore satisfactory oxygenation and ventilation have been taken
- first line inotrope as an infusion centrally or peripherally in fluid resistant septic shock
- anaphylaxis

In cardiac arrest with non-shockable rhythms, adrenaline should be given as soon as circulatory access has been achieved, as early administration is associated with better outcomes. In shockable rhythms, adrenaline should be given after the third defibrillation and then following alternate shocks after that (e.g. following the third shock, then following the fifth shock etc.).

Dosage
In cardiorespiratory arrest (shockable/non-shockable rhythms, or bradycardia) with decompensated circulatory failure, the dose of adrenaline is 10 mcg kg^{-1} (or 0.1 mL kg^{-1} of 1:10 000 solution) IV or IO. This is repeated every 3–5 min as necessary.

IM adrenaline dose for anaphylaxis
< 6 months
100–150 microgram IM (0.1–0.15 mL of 1 mg mL (1:1000) adrenaline

6 months–6 years
150 microgram IM (0.15 mL of 1 mg mL (1:1000) adrenaline

6–12 years
300 microgram IM (0.3 mL of 1 mg mL (1:1000) adrenaline

12+ years
500 microgram IM (0.5 mL of 1 mg mL (1:1000) adrenaline

Actions
Adrenaline is an endogenous, directly acting sympathomimetic amine with both alpha and beta-adrenergic activity. In the dose used in resuscitation, adrenaline produces vasoconstriction, which results in increased cerebral and coronary perfusion pressure. It also increases myocardial contractility and may facilitate defibrillation success.

Adrenaline frequently causes tachycardia and may produce or exacerbate ventricular ectopics.

Higher doses of adrenaline administered by the vascular route are not recommended routinely as they do not improve survival or neurological outcome after cardiorespiratory arrest.

Amiodarone

Indications for use
Refractory ventricular fibrillation (VF) or pulseless ventricular tachycardia (pVT). If VF or pVT persists after the 3rd defibrillation shock, a dose of amiodarone should be given as well as adrenaline. This can be repeated after the 5th shock if defibrillation is still unsuccessful.

Dosage
5 mg kg^{-1}.

Actions
Amiodarone is a membrane-stabilising anti-arrhythmic medication that increases the duration of the action potential and refractory period in both atrial and ventricular myocardium.

Precautions
Amiodarone should be given as a pre-filled syringe preparation or diluted in 5% glucose. Ideally, it should be administered via a central vascular (IV or IO) route as it can cause thrombophlebitis. If it has to be given peripherally it should be liberally flushed with 0.9% sodium chloride or 5% glucose.

Important to note
In patients with a pulse, amiodarone may be used to treat tachyarrhythmias (SVT, VT). In this scenario, it must be infused over 20 min or greater; this is because severe hypotension, bradycardia and even cardiac arrest may occur with faster infusion rates.

Sodium bicarbonate

This is not a first-line resuscitation medication. Studies have shown that the routine use of sodium bicarbonate does not improve outcome. Whilst the routine use of sodium bicarbonate is not recommended, it may be considered in prolonged arrest and it has a specific role in the management of hyperkalaemia and the arrhythmias associated with tricyclic antidepressant or some inborn errors of metabolism.

Dosage

The initial dose is 1 mmol kg^{-1}. This equates to 1 mL kg^{-1} of 8.4% solution, although in newborns and infants < 3 months, the weaker concentration (i.e. 4.2%) solution should be used to limit the osmotic load.

The decision to give further doses should be based on blood gas analysis.

Adenosine

Indications for use

Adenosine is used in the management of SVT as it impairs accessory bundle re-entry at the AV node.

Adenosine is rapidly metabolised by red blood cells, and its half-life is only 10 s. Therefore, it should be injected rapidly and as close to the heart as possible (via a central or upper limb peripheral intravenous route) and immediately followed by a rapid bolus of 0.9% sodium chloride. Unfortunately, it is often seen to be ineffective when given via IO access in the tibia.

Continuous cardiac monitoring with printout is required so that a cardiologist can interpret the initial rhythm later and to monitor the effect of adenosine, which may be diagnostic.

Dosage (BNFc)
Neonates

Initially 150 mcg kg^{-1} then increased in steps of 50-100 mcg kg^{-1} every 1–2 min if required; dose to be repeated until tachycardia terminated or maximum single dose of 300 mcg kg^{-1} given

Child 1–11 months

Initially 150 mcg kg^{-1}, then increased in steps of 50–100 mcg kg^{-1} every 1–2 min if required; dose to be repeated until tachycardia terminated or maximum single dose of 500 mcg kg^{-1} given

Child 1–11 years

Initially 100 mcg kg^{-1} then increased in steps of 50–100 mcg kg every 1–2 min if required; dose to be repeated until tachycardia terminated or maximum single dose of 500 mcg kg^{-1} given (max 12 mg)

Child 12–17 years

Initially 3 mg, followed by 6 mg after 1–2 min if required, followed by 12 mg after 1–2 min if required

Precautions

Adenosine should be used with caution in asthmatics (as it can invoke severe bronchospasm) and children who have undergone a heart transplant.

Glucose

Indications for use

Documented hypoglycaemia. Neonatal, child and adult data show that both hyper and hypoglycaemia are associated with worse outcomes after cardiorespiratory arrest. Plasma glucose concentrations should be monitored closely in any ill or injured child, including after cardiorespiratory arrest. Do not give glucose-containing fluids during CPR except for the treatment of hypoglycaemia.

The clinical signs of hypoglycaemia and shock may have similarities, (i.e. hypotension, tachycardia, decreased peripheral perfusion and sweating), so always check the blood glucose in any child with these symptoms or any child with coma or seizures (which may also be symptoms of hypoglycaemia).

Dosage

200 mg kg^{-1} (2 mL kg^{-1} of 10% glucose solution)

Newborn

2.5 mL kg^{-1} of 10% glucose solution

Re-checking the blood glucose value should be performed shortly afterwards (e.g. 2–5 min following administration) to determine if further dosages are required.

Atropine

Indications for use

Bradycardia resulting from vagal stimulation. There is no evidence that atropine has any benefit in asphyxial bradycardia or asystole and its routine use has been removed from the advanced life support algorithms.

Dosage
Up to 11 years of age

20 mcg kg^{-1}

Child 12–17 years

300–600 mcg (larger doses may be used in emergencies)

These dosages may be repeated but, once the vagus nerve has been fully blocked, there is no further beneficial effect.

Actions

Atropine blocks the effect of the vagus nerve on the sinoatrial (SA) and atrioventricular (AV) nodes, increasing sinus automaticity, facilitating AV node conduction and increasing heart rate. The functions of the vagus nerve include pupillary constriction, contraction of the gut and production of salivary and gastrointestinal secretions. During resuscitation, atropine may be of benefit in treating bradycardia which accompanies actions that result in vagal stimulation such as laryngoscopy.

06: **Summary learning**

Intraosseous access is the circulatory route of choice in cardiorespiratory arrest and decompensated circulatory failure.

Fluid resuscitation starts with 10 mL kg^{-1} boluses.

After each fluid bolus, the child's condition must be reassessed.

The role of medications is secondary to effective ventilation and chest compressions (and, if indicated, defibrillation) in cardiorespiratory arrest.

The main medication used in cardiorespiratory arrest is IV or IO adrenaline, which can be repeated as necessary every 3–5 min.

Amiodarone is used in refractory VF or pVT after the 3rd and 5th shock.

My key take-home messages from this chapter are:

Further reading

Maitland K, Kiguli S, Opoka RO, Engoru C, Olupot-Olupot P, Akech SO, Nyeko R, Mtove G, Reyburn H, Lang T, Brent B, Evans JA, Tibenderana JK, Crawley J,Russell EC, Levin M, Babiker AG, Gibb DM; FEAST Trial Group. Mortality after fluid bolus in African children with severe infection. NEJM. 2011, Jun 30;364(26):2483-95.

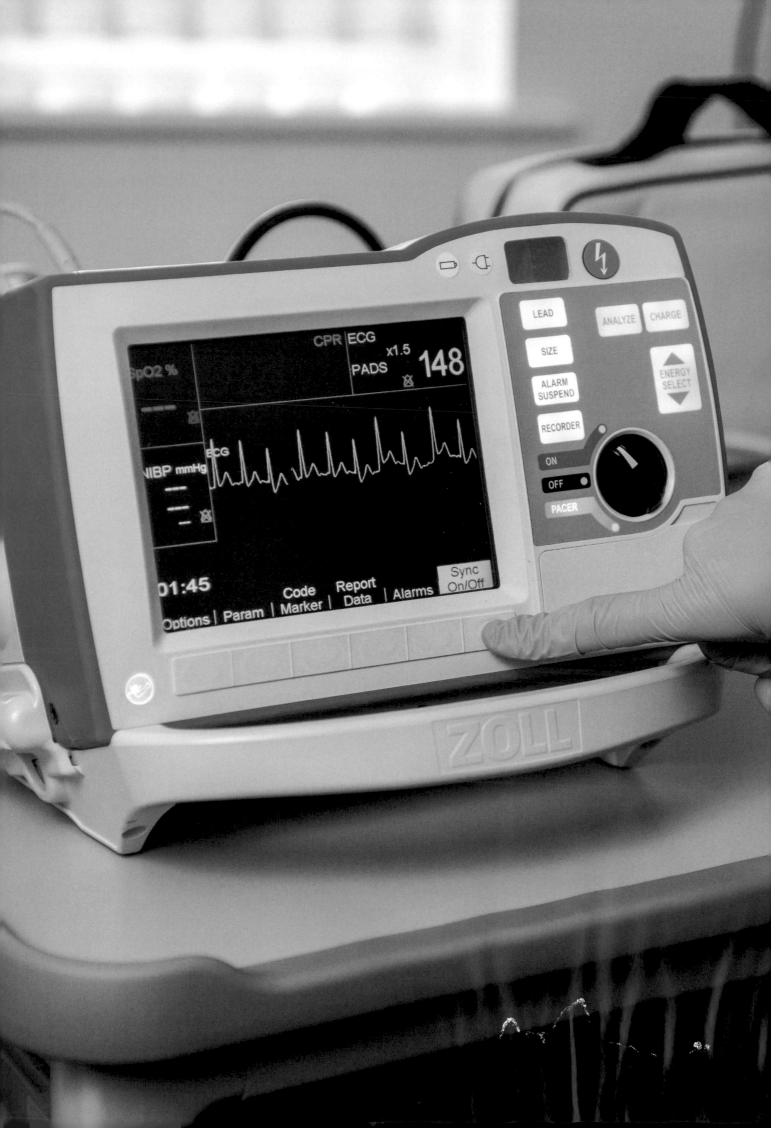

Rhythm recognition

ECG monitoring

Once optimal ventilation and oxygenation have been established, all seriously ill children should have their ECG monitored continuously via lead II, and at least one 12-lead ECG should be performed.

This facilitates the observation of heart rate and rhythm changes, which are important indicators of the response to treatments or the evolution of the disease process. Normal heart rates vary for physiological reasons (e.g. pain, pyrexia and wakefulness), and with age (Table 7.1).

Acute illness in children can result in cardiac arrhythmias. Less frequently, the cardiac arrhythmia may be the precipitant for the episode of acute illness. In these cases, there is commonly an underlying cardiac anatomic anomaly or reason for electrolyte disturbance causing abnormal cardiac electrical conductivity.

Examples include:

- acquired cardiac disease (e.g. cardiomyopathy, myocarditis)
- congenital heart disease or following cardiac surgery
- electrolyte disturbances (e.g. renal disease).

Additionally, some medications in therapeutic or toxic amounts may also cause arrhythmias (e.g. digoxin, beta-blockers, tricyclic antidepressants).

By monitoring the ECG, it is possible to detect those arrhythmias that are (or have the potential to become) life-threatening.

Table 7.1 Heart rate ranges (beats min⁻¹)

Age	Mean	Awake	Deep sleep
Newborn – 3 months	140	85–205	80–140
3 months – 2 years	130	100–180	75–160
2–10 years	80	60–140	60–90
> 10 years	75	60–100	50–90

Acute illness in children can result in cardiac arrhythmias

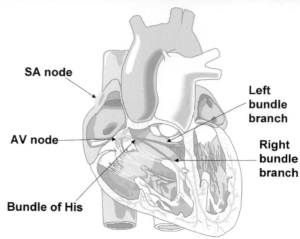

Figure 7.2   Electrical conduction through the heart

Basic electrocardiography

The ECG trace represents electrical activity within the heart, not the effectiveness of myocardial contraction or tissue perfusion. The child's clinical status needs to be considered alongside the ECG trace: treat the patient, not the monitor.

When evaluating the ECG, possible artefacts may occur; detachment of ECG electrodes or leads can simulate asystole, whilst vibrations transmitted to the leads (e.g. during patient transportation) can mimic ventricular fibrillation (VF).

A normal ECG complex consists of a P wave, a QRS complex and a T wave (Figure 7.1).

Looking at an ECG rhythm strip

Standard ECG paper is composed of small squares; when the paper speed is 25 mm sec^{-1} each square represents 0.04 s. The larger squares are 5mm in length on the ECG paper and represent 0.2 s. The heart rate can be calculated by counting the number of QRS complexes in 6 s (30 large squares) and multiplying this number by 10.

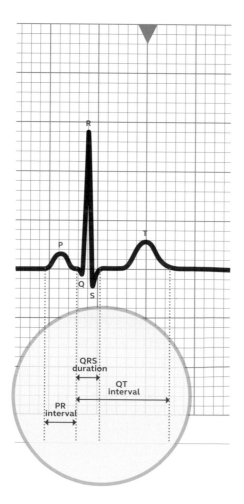

Figure 7.1   The normal ECG complex

The ECG

The electrical impulse normally starts from the sinoatrial node in the right atrium and stimulates atrial contraction. As the impulse moves through the atrium to the Atrioventricular node, a positive deflection is seen on the ECG rhythm strip known as the P wave. P waves are normally 2 small squares lasting 0.08–0.1 s on the ECG paper and represent electrical depolarisation of the atria. The time taken for depolarisation to pass through the atria, atrioventricular (AV) node and His-Purkinje system to the ventricles (Figure 7.2) is represented by the P–R interval (lasting 0.08–0.15 s (2–4 small squares on the ECG paper)). A prolonged P–R interval suggests a degree of heart block.

The QRS complex represents depolarisation of the ventricles which stimulates the right and left ventricles to contract. This is seen on the ECG as the large QRS complex (lasting around 0.08–0.12 s (2–3 small squares on the ECG paper)). Abnormalities in conduction pathways through the ventricles can cause abnormalities to ventricular conduction. This may be seen as widening of the QRS complex. The ST segment and the T wave represent ventricular repolarisation, in preparation for the next impulse. A prolonged QT interval (a delay between the beginning of ventricular depolarisation and repolarisation) is a risk factor for arrhythmias and sudden death.

It is important to remember that the ECG complex relates to electrical activity of the heart, not muscular contraction. Therefore, always assess and treat the patient not the monitor.

Cardiac rhythm disturbances

The approach to managing a child with a cardiac rhythm disturbance is summarised in Figure 7.3. This approach is based on determining the following four factors:

1. Presence or absence of circulation (i.e. a central pulse and other 'signs of life').
2. Clinical status – compensated (haemodynamically stable) or decompensated (haemodynamically unstable).
3. Heart rate (bradycardia or tachycardia).
4. Width of QRS complexes on ECG (i.e. narrow or broad).

Paediatric cardiac arrhythmias

Assess with ABCDE approach – recognise and treat reversible causes
Oxygen if SpO$_2$ < 94%, respiratory rate, heart rate, CRT, cardiac monitoring, blood pressure, vascular access, AVPU

Signs of circulation?

NO → Follow **ADVANCED LIFE SUPPORT ALGORITHM**

YES

Compensated
Normal LOC, +/- respiratory distress and signs of circulatory compromise, BP > 5th centile*

Monitor for clinical deterioration and seek expert help

Treat the cause:
If bradycardia, consider oxygenation and vagal tone
If SVT, consider vagal manoeuvres
Reassess
Consider adenosine

Decompensated – seek expert help

Signs of vital organ perfusion compromise:
Reduced LOC, tachypnoea, bradycardia /tachycardia, BP < 5th centile*, CRT > 2 secs, weak or impalpable peripheral pulses

Bradycardia

< 1 year < 80 min^{-1}
> 1 year < 60 min^{-1}

Optimal oxygenation with positive pressure ventilation if required

If unconscious and HR < 60 min^{-1} despite oxygenation, start chest compressions

No response to oxygenation:
If vagal stimulation possible cause – atropine
If no response to oxygenation or atropine consider adrenaline
Pacing – very rarely required and guided by aetiology.

Tachycardia

Narrow complex

Sinus tachycardia
Infant typically 180–220 min^{-1}
Child typically 160–180 min^{-1}
Gradual onset

Treat the cause:
Physiological response:
– Crying
– Exercise
– Anxiety/fear
– Pain

Identify precipitant
Compensatory mechanism:
– Respiratory/circulatory failure
– Hypovolaemia
– Sepsis
– Anaemia

SVT
Infant > 220 min^{-1}
Child > 180 min^{-1}
Abrupt onset

Synchronised cardioversion with appropriate sedation + analgesia (e.g. IM/intranasal ketamine if delay in IV access)
Chemical cardioversion may be 1st choice if suitable IV access is in place and delay in synchronised cardioversion.
Adenosine
Consider amiodarone before 3rd shock

Broad complex

VT
Could be VT or SVT, if unsure treat as VT

If conscious:
Synchronised cardioversion with appropriate sedation + analgesia (e.g. IM/intranasal ketamine if delay in IV access, *do not delay cardioversion*).

If unconscious:
Immediate synchronised cardioversion
Consider amiodarone before 3rd shock

Drug	Atropine	Adrenaline	Adenosine	Amiodarone	Synchronised cardioversion	Magnesium
Treatment	**Up to 11 years:** 20 mcg kg^{-1}. **12–17 years:** 300–600 mcg, larger doses may be used in emergency.	**For bradycardia:** 10 mcg kg^{-1} repeat if necessary.	**Up to 1 year:** 150 mcg kg^{-1}, increase 50–100 mcg kg^{-1} every 1–2 min. Maximum single dose: Neonates 300 mcg kg^{-1}, Infants 500 mcg kg^{-1}) **1–11 years:** 100 mcg kg^{-1} increase 50–100 mcg kg^{-1} every 1–2 min. Maximum single dose: 500 mcg kg^{-1} (max. 12 mg). **12–17 years:** 3 mg IV, if required increase to 6 mg after 1–2 min, then 12 mg after 1–2 min	5 mg kg^{-1} – by SLOW IV infusion (> 20 min) before 3rd cardioversion in discussion with paediatric cardiologist/expert	With appropriate sedation + analgesia (e.g. IM/intranasal Ketamine if delay in IV access + airway management) – IV access attempts must not delay cardioversion **1st shock:** 1 J kg^{-1} **2nd shock:** 2 J kg^{-1}, consider up to 4 J kg^{-1}	25–50 mg kg^{-1} Maximum per dose 2 g to be given over 10–15 min, may be repeated once if necessary, in Torsades de pointes VT

Age	*Systolic BP 5th centile mmHg
1 month	50
1 year	70
5 years	75
10 years	80

Figure 7.3   Managing the child with a cardiac arrhythmia

1. Presence of central pulse

Adopt the ABCDE approach and quickly establish the absence or presence of cardiac output (i.e. signs of life and a palpable central pulse).

Absent pulse

The absence of 'signs of life' and no palpable central pulse indicates cardiorespiratory arrest. BLS should be started immediately. The rhythms associated with cardiorespiratory arrest are:

- asystole (or severe bradycardia, < 60 min^{-1} with signs of inadequate perfusion)
- pulseless electrical activity (PEA)
- ventricular fibrillation (VF)
- pulseless ventricular tachycardia (pVT).

The commonest cardiorespiratory arrest arrhythmia in paediatrics is asystole (generally preceded by progressive bradycardia). The term PEA describes the situation where there is organised electrical activity displayed on the ECG monitor but no cardiac output. The principles of managing both asystole and PEA are the provision of effective CPR, early administration of adrenaline and the treatment of any reversible causes. Both VF and pVT are less common in children but more likely in those with underlying cardiac disease (congenital or acquired). The priority of management in these arrhythmias is effective CPR and rapid defibrillation. VF and pVT may also occur as a secondary rhythm during reperfusion of the myocardium during a cardiorespiratory arrest.

Any possible causes (or aggravating factors) that have a specific treatment, including reversible causes, must be considered during all cardiorespiratory arrests. The management of cardiorespiratory arrest arrhythmias is outlined in Chapter 9.

Pulse present

If there is a central pulse present, determine whether or not the child is compensated (haemodynamically stable) or decompensated (haemodynamically unstable).

2. Clinical status

Compensated circulatory failure

The child with compensated circulatory failure, who is conscious and haemodynamically stable, must be monitored, including an ECG. If the ECG displays an arrhythmia, the child may need treatment, but it is reasonable to await expert help such as from a paediatric cardiologist. Preparations should be made to intervene should the child deteriorate and become decompensated. (See Chapter 2.)

Decompensated circulatory failure

The child who is decompensated (haemodynamically unstable) should be monitored and, if the ECG displays a life-threatening arrhythmia, the immediate interventions that may be required are outlined below. Urgent expert help must also be sought. This should include an anaesthetist as sedation or anaesthesia may be required to manage a conscious child requiring cardioversion.

3. Heart rate

Both bradycardia and tachycardia are relatively common in paediatrics. Their typical defining heart rates are listed in Table 7.2.

Table 7.2   Typical bradycardia and tachycardia heart rates

Age	Bradycardia	Tachycardia
< 1 year	< 80* beats min^{-1}	> 180 beats min^{-1}
> 1 year	< 60 beats min^{-1}	> 160 beats min^{-1}
*although 80 min^{-1} is defining rate for bradycardia in an infant, chest compressions are not indicated until the heart rate is < 60 min^{-1} (with signs of inadequate perfusion).		

Bradycardia

Bradycardia may be due to hypoxia, acidosis and respiratory or circulatory failure, or it may be a pre-terminal event prior to cardiorespiratory arrest.

A bradycardic child with signs of decompensation or a child with a rapidly dropping heart rate associated with poor systemic perfusion requires immediate oxygenation (airway opening, 100% oxygen administration and positive pressure ventilation as necessary). If the heart rate remains < 60 min^{-1} (all ages) and the child is unconscious with decompensated circulatory failure, chest compressions must also be started. The cause of the bradycardia must be sought and treatment directed at the underlying cause.

By far, the commonest causes of bradycardia in infants and children are hypoxia and vagal stimulation. Less commonly, hypothermia and hypoglycaemia can slow conduction through cardiac tissues and result in bradycardia. Infants and children with a history of heart surgery are at increased risk of damage to the AV node or other parts of the conduction system.

Atropine is indicated when increased vagal tone is the cause of the bradycardia (e.g. induced by tracheal intubation or suctioning). Otherwise, adrenaline is the medication of choice but only once oxygenation has been restored, and the HR remains < 60 min^{-1} with circulatory failure. Very occasionally, in a child with congenital heart disease, the bradycardia is due to complete heart block, and emergency cardiac pacing is required. Pacing is not

Figure 7.4 Bradycardia

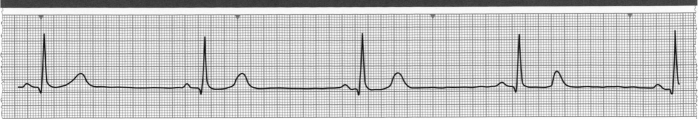

Figure 7.5 Sinus tachycardia rhythm strip

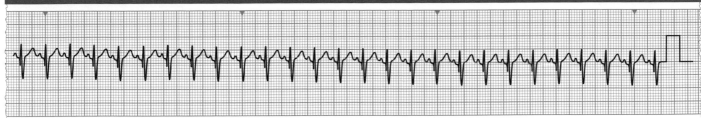

Figure 7.6 Supraventricular tachycardia rhythm strip

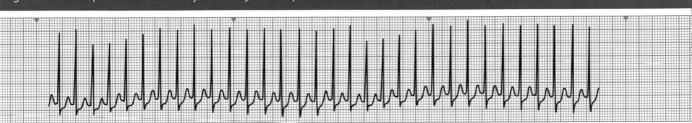

indicated and is ineffective in children with bradycardia secondary to hypoxic/ischaemic myocardial insult or respiratory failure.

Tachycardia

An elevated heart rate is frequently the normal physiological response to anxiety, pain or pyrexia. This is sinus tachycardia (ST) and is managed by treating the primary cause.

Other causes of ST include:

- respiratory conditions; early hypoxia, hypercapnia, obstructed airway and pneumothorax
- circulatory conditions; hypovolaemia, cardiac failure, anaphylaxis, sepsis or pulmonary hypertension
- miscellaneous causes; drugs, seizures.

The other cause of tachycardia is an arrhythmia, either supraventricular tachycardia (SVT) or ventricular tachycardia (VT).

Of these, SVT is far more common in children. The priority of management is to establish whether the child is stable or if they are displaying signs of circulatory decompensation. If the child is in a compensated state, expert help should be sought for definitive management.

The child who has decompensated circulatory failure requires chemical or electrical cardioversion whilst their ABCDE is continually assessed and appropriately supported.

4. Width of QRS complexes

In children with a tachycardia, the most important thing to establish is whether this is ST or an abnormal rhythm (tachyarrhythmia). The history and clinical examination are key in determining this. The ECG features and width of the QRS complexes can also be helpful, but it is always the child's clinical status that determines the urgency of management, regardless of the type of arrhythmia.

Narrow QRS complex tachycardia

Both ST (Figure 7.5) and SVT (Figure 7.6) have narrow QRS complexes making it potentially difficult to differentiate between them. The clinical and ECG differences that help to make this distinction are listed in Table 7.3.

Table 7.3 Distinguishing features between ST and SVT

	ST	SVT
Onset and termination	Gradual	Abrupt
History	Clues (e.g. pyrexia, fluid or blood loss)	Non-specific Previous arrhythmia
Heart rate (beats min^{-1})	Infant < 220 min^{-1} Child < 180 min^{-1}	Infant > 220 min^{-1} Child > 180 min^{-1}
P wave	Present and normal (NB not clearly seen at heart rates > 200 min^{-1})	Absent or abnormal
Beat-to-beat variability (R–R)	Yes – can be altered with stimulation	None

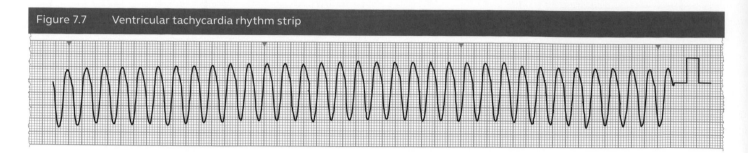

Figure 7.7   Ventricular tachycardia rhythm strip

Broad QRS complex tachycardia

In children, broad complex tachycardia is uncommon and is usually due to an SVT. However, if uncertain, carefully consider VT (Figure 7.7) as this has more immediately serious consequences if inadequately treated (i.e. it can deteriorate to pVT or VF).

VT is usually found in a child who has an underlying cardiac disease (congenital or acquired) or after certain drug ingestions.

VT is a broad complex, regular rhythm. The P waves are either absent or unrelated to the QRS complexes (Figure 7.7). It can present with or without a pulse; pulseless VT (pVT) is managed in the same manner as VF (i.e. with CPR and urgent defibrillation).

Management of VT with a pulse

The management of VT with a pulse involves urgent expert consultation, as it has the potential to rapidly deteriorate to pVT or VF. The ongoing management of these children may involve electrical cardioversion or chemical cardioversion (usually with amiodarone). An anaesthetist or paediatric intensivist should be contacted in addition to a cardiologist as amiodarone can cause hypotension and may result in rapid circulatory decompensation, and if electrical cardioversion is required, anaesthesia may be necessary.

Supraventricular tachycardia

SVT is the most common primary cardiac arrhythmia observed in children. It is a paroxysmal, regular rhythm with narrow QRS complexes caused by a re-entry mechanism through an accessory pathway or the atrioventricular conduction system. A heart rate of > 220 min^{-1} in infants or > 180 min^{-1} in children older than one year is highly suggestive of SVT. The other features that differentiate SVT from ST are listed in Table 7.3.

Management of SVT

Once a diagnosis of SVT is made, the child's clinical status will determine the management. As described previously, a child with compensated circulatory status should be referred for expert help. Treatment may include vagal manoeuvres, adenosine or cardioversion.

Vagal manoeuvres

In infants and small children, this can be performed by soaking a flannel in ice cold water and then placing it briefly over their face. In cooperative children, a Valsalva manoeuvre can be induced by asking the child to blow through a drinking straw. A variation on this is to blow through the outlet of a syringe in an effort to expel the plunger.

Adenosine

If intravascular access is already established in a conscious, compensated child with SVT, chemical cardioversion with adenosine may be possible. Adenosine should be given rapidly via a vein as close to the heart as possible, as it is metabolised by red blood cells as soon as it enters the bloodstream. It is very helpful to have an ECG rhythm strip running during administration as this may help in diagnosis when reviewed by a paediatric cardiologist.

Doses: see Chapter 6.

Cardioversion

The procedure for undertaking synchronised electrical cardioversion is described in Chapter 8. It is the procedure of choice for decompensated children with tachyarrhythmia, particularly if they are unconscious. Analgesia and sedation with airway management by an experienced provider, preferably an anaesthetist, will be required if the child is conscious (e.g. intramuscular or intranasal ketamine can be considered if the child has no intravenous access). Most importantly, cardioversion should not be unnecessarily delayed by intravenous access attempts. The first shock should be delivered at the energy level of 1 J kg^{-1}, and the second (if required) at 2 J kg^{-1}. Clinicians can consider increasing to 4 J kg^{-1} under expert guidance. Additionally, if the tachyarrhythmia fails to convert after the second shock, amiodarone infusion over > 20 min may be recommended before further shocks are delivered; again, this should ideally be under the guidance of a paediatric cardiologist or paediatric intensivist.

07: **Summary learning**

Life-threatening cardiac arrhythmias are more frequently the result, rather than the cause, of acute illness.

The child's clinical status dictates management priorities – treat the patient, not the monitor.

The cause of the arrhythmia should be sought and treated.

My key take-home messages from this chapter are:

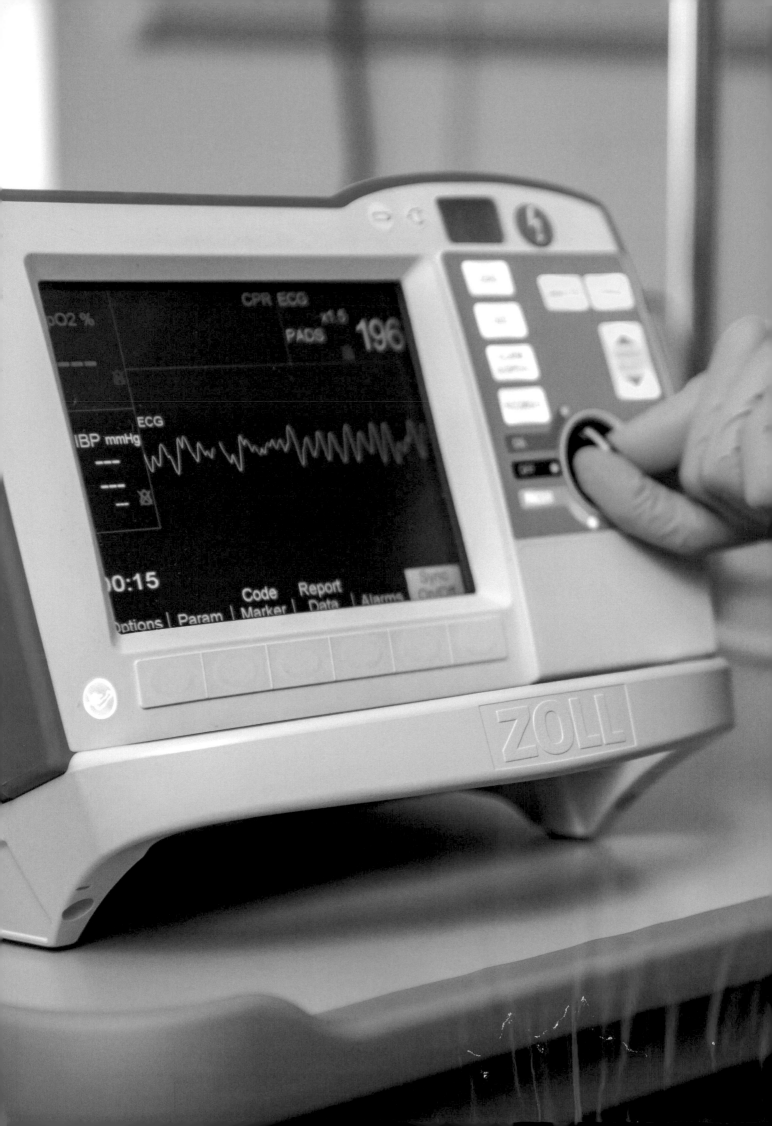

Defibrillation and cardioversion

Incidence of shockable arrhythmias

Although the initial rhythm in a paediatric cardiorespiratory arrest is far more likely to be asystole or pulseless electrical activity (PEA) than ventricular fibrillation (VF) or pulseless ventricular tachycardia (pVT), a shockable rhythm is present in up to 27% of paediatric in-hospital arrests at some point during the resuscitation. When a shockable rhythm is present, the likelihood of a successful outcome is critically dependent on rapid, safe defibrillation.

A defibrillator can also be used in the management of a child with circulatory compromise due to VT with a pulse or supraventricular tachycardia (SVT) (Chapter 7). In these situations, the machine is used to perform synchronised DC (direct current) cardioversion, which is also described in this chapter.

A shockable rhythm is present in up to 27% of paediatric in-hospital arrests at some point during the resuscitation

When a shockable rhythm is present, the likelihood of a successful outcome is critically dependent on rapid, safe defibrillation

Defibrillation

Defibrillation is the generic term used to describe the procedure of passing an electrical current across the myocardium with the intention of inducing global myocardial depolarisation and restoring organised spontaneous electrical activity. This electrical current may be delivered asynchronously when there is no cardiac output (in VF or pVT), or it may be synchronised with the R wave when there is an output (in SVT or VT with a pulse), the latter being called cardioversion.

The energy dosage should cause minimal myocardial injury. The electrical current delivered to the heart depends on the selected energy (in joules) and the resistance to current flow (thoracic impedance). If the impedance is high, the energy requirement will be increased.

Factors determining thoracic impedance

The factors that potentially affect thoracic impedance and therefore the energy required, include:

- defibrillator pads/paddles size
- interface between pads/paddles and the child's skin
- positioning of the pads/paddles on the chest wall
- chest wall thickness and obesity.

Types of defibrillators

Defibrillators are either automatic (i.e. automated external defibrillators (AEDs)) or manually operated. They may be capable of delivering either monophasic or biphasic shocks. AEDs are pre-set for all parameters, including the energy dose.

Manual defibrillators capable of delivering the full range of energy requirements for newborns through to adults must be available within all healthcare facilities caring for children at risk of cardiorespiratory arrest. In children requiring cardioversion (e.g. a child with circulatory failure from SVT) a manual defibrillator should be used as AEDs do not have synchronisation technology.

Biphasic defibrillators

There are various types of biphasic waveform, but there is no data to support one being superior to another. There is, however, good evidence that biphasic defibrillators are more effective than monophasic ones. A biphasic defibrillator delivers a current that flows in a positive direction and then in reverse for a specified duration. First shock efficacy for long-lasting VF/pVT is better with biphasic than monophasic waveforms. Biphasic waves also appear to cause less post-shock cardiac dysfunction.

Paddles or pads?

Manual defibrillation is now more commonly performed using self-adhesive pads (i.e. 'hands-free' defibrillation) rather than using manual defibrillator paddles. Self-adhesive pads are safe, effective and generally preferable to defibrillator paddles. A major advantage of using self-adhesive pads is that they allow the rescuer to defibrillate from a safe distance, rather than having to lean across the patient; this is particularly important when access to the patient is restricted in a confined space. They deliver the shock more rapidly and with less interruption to CPR as the machine can be charged whilst chest compressions are in progress. Some self-adhesive pads have a sensor attached which measures rate, depth and recoil of chest compressions so that the rescuer can monitor the quality of CPR delivered.

Position of self-adhesive pads

Self-adhesive pads should be placed on the child's chest in a position that 'brackets' the heart to facilitate the flow of electrical current across it.

The anterior-posterior (A-P) pad position (Figure 8.1); place the anterior pad on the lower half of the chest slightly to the left of the sternum and the posterior pad between the scapulae. The A-P position may be preferred in infants because of the size of the chest. In older children, where the chest may be larger, and it is believed CPR will be interrupted and defibrillation delayed, in order to place the posterior pad the antero-lateral pad position may be preferred.

The antero-lateral (A-L) pad position (Figure 8.2): one pad is placed just below the right clavicle to the right of the sternum and the other in the mid-axillary line on the left of the chest in the V5–V6 position of a 12-lead ECG.

There is no evidence to suggest one position is superior to the other; however, it is important that the defibrillator pads must not touch. If defibrillation pads touch, the energy arcs across the chest from pad to pad and not through the chest.

A selection of appropriate pads relating to the child's size/age may also be necessary, 8–12 cm is recommended for use in children and 4.5 cm for infants, although this varies between manufacturers. The pads should be smoothed onto the child's chest, ensuring that no air is trapped underneath, as this will increase impedance and reduce the efficiency of the defibrillation shock. Although the pads have a diagram of their correct positioning on the chest, it does not matter if they have been reversed. Therefore, if they have accidentally been placed the wrong way round, they should be left in place and not repositioned. Repositioning results in time-wasting, and the self-adhesive pads may stick less effectively.

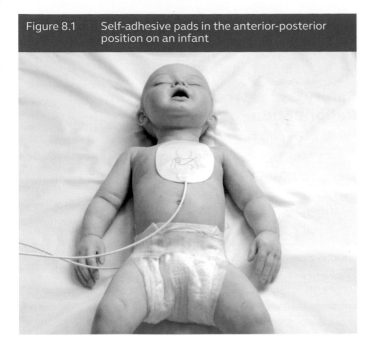

Figure 8.1 Self-adhesive pads in the anterior-posterior position on an infant

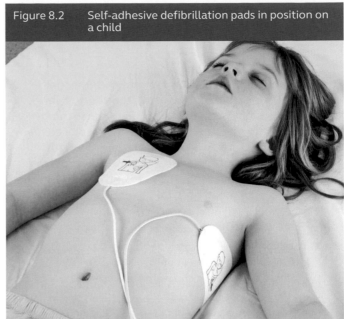

Figure 8.2 Self-adhesive defibrillation pads in position on a child

Energy levels

Manual defibrillators

Manual defibrillators (Figure 8.3) have several advantages over AEDs and therefore, must be readily available in all healthcare settings where children at risk of cardiorespiratory arrest may be cared for, even when AEDs are located nearby. The advantages include:

- ability to alter energy levels

- trained operators can diagnose arrhythmias and, when appropriate, deliver shocks more rapidly (with AEDs this diagnosis must await the results of the machine's rhythm analysis)

- additional facilities permit other treatments (e.g. synchronised cardioversion or external pacing).

Note: when using a manual defibrillator an energy dose of 4 J per kg body weight (4 J kg^{-1}) should be used for all shocks. In a large child, adult doses should not be exceeded.

Automated external defibrillators

These machines are now widely available including through Public Access Defibrillation (PAD) schemes as fully or semi-automated devices (Figure 8.4). They are safe, reliable and sophisticated and are increasingly used by health professionals and lay rescuers.

If there is any likelihood of use in infants and small children check with the manufacturer that the machine is suitable. Machines with paediatric attenuation devices are preferable.

The AED will analyse the patient's ECG rhythm, determine whether a defibrillation shock is indicated and facilitate the delivery of a shock. In the semi-automated models, follow the AED prompts and press the relevant button.

Some of the models available to healthcare professionals have the facility for the operator to override the AED and deliver a shock independently of any prompting by the machine.

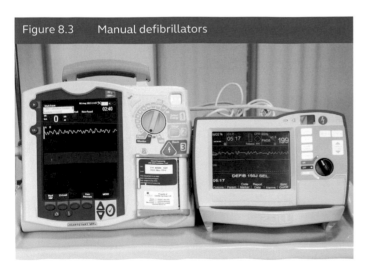

Figure 8.3 Manual defibrillators

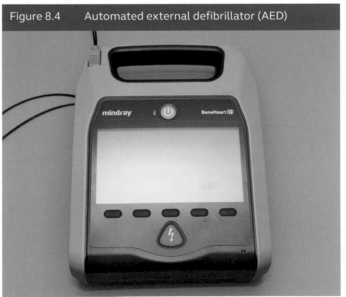

Figure 8.4 Automated external defibrillator (AED)

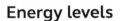

The main advantages of AEDs are that they recognise VF and pVT shockable rhythms, and therefore, a shock can be delivered by a lay-person. They are also relatively cheap and lightweight and have therefore replaced many manual defibrillators. Available AEDs have been tested extensively against libraries of adult ECG rhythms and in trials in adults and children. They are extremely accurate in rhythm recognition in both adults and children. The voice prompts from the AED must be followed to ensure safe, effective practice.

- If a child > 8 years requires defibrillation, standard adult AED energy levels can be used.
- If a child < 8 years requires defibrillation, and there is no manual defibrillator available, an AED can be used. The AED should ideally be equipped with a dose attenuator, which decreases the delivered energy to a lower, more appropriate dosage (generally 50–75 J).

If such an AED is unavailable in an emergency situation, then a standard AED with adult energy levels may be used. The upper dose limit for safe defibrillation is unknown, but higher doses than the previously recommended 4 J kg^{-1} have defibrillated children effectively and without significant adverse effects. Higher doses are acceptable because defibrillation is the only effective treatment for VF/pVT.

Infants have a much lower incidence of shockable rhythms, and good quality CPR is the treatment priority. If an infant is in a shockable rhythm and a manual machine is not available, the use of an AED (preferably with attenuator) may be considered.

Minimal interruption to chest compressions

Every time chest compressions are interrupted, even for a brief period, a low flow state is created where coronary artery and cerebral perfusion pressures fall dramatically. Several chest compressions are required to return these pressures to optimum levels. Interruptions can be minimised during defibrillation by:

- Good team communication and coordination.
- Charging the defibrillator whilst chest compressions are ongoing during the shockable arm of the ALS algorithm.
- Minimising the delay between stopping chest compressions and the delivery of shocks or checking for signs of life at the end of 2 min cycles (< 5 s is ideal).
- Resuming chest compressions immediately after the delivery of a shock with no check of either the monitor or patient.

Safety issues when undertaking defibrillation

The safety of the rescuers, as well as that of the child, is paramount. The following factors must be considered.

Oxygen

All free-flowing oxygen delivery devices (O_2 masks or nasal cannulae) must be removed from the immediate area and placed at least one metre from the child. If the child is being ventilated via a sealed advanced airway (SGA, TT), the ventilation bag or ventilator tubing can be left connected if it forms part of a closed circuit. If the circuit is disconnected for whatever reason, the devices must be placed at least one metre away from the child.

Dry surfaces

Any wet clothing should be removed from the immediate area. The surface the child is laid on, and the child's chest should be wiped dry if necessary before shock delivery.

Contact with patient

The person delivering the shock must ensure that neither they nor any other rescuers/relatives are in direct or indirect contact with the child during shock delivery.

There should be no contact between the pads and any metal objects (e.g. jewellery) or items such as transdermal medication or diathermy pads.

Operator instructions

Familiarity with the defibrillator being used increases safety for all the team and operator efficiency. Operators must also ensure that they issue clear instructions to the rest of the team/bystanders to facilitate safe practice throughout the procedure.

Sequence of actions for defibrillation

If the ALS rescuer is first on scene, the entire BLS sequence needs to be followed. If, however, the rescuer is part of a response team arriving to find BLS already ongoing, they should reconfirm cardiorespiratory arrest taking no more than 5 s to do so. Having confirmed cardiorespiratory arrest, CPR should be started (or restarted) while the team member operating the defibrillator prepares as follows:

1. Confirms presence of shockable rhythm (VF/pVT) via self-adhesive/monitoring pads or ECG monitor during a brief pause in chest compressions.
2. Instructs the team to resume chest compressions, preferably using a sensor allowing CPR feedback and metronomic support if available.

3. Selects the appropriate energy (4 J kg⁻¹).

4. Warns all team members other than the individual performing the chest compressions to "stand clear" and remove any oxygen delivery device as appropriate.

5. Charges the defibrillator to the required energy level whilst chest compressions are ongoing.

6. Once the defibrillator is charged, tell the team member doing the chest compressions to "stand clear"; when clear and after confirming continued VF/pVT, delivers the shock.

7. Without reassessing the rhythm or feeling for a pulse, instructs team to restart CPR starting with chest compressions. The team should then continue CPR for 2 min; the team leader resumes coordination of the team and prepares for the next pause in CPR. If VF/pVT persists after 2 min of CPR, deliver a second shock/subsequent shocks.

Further management of shockable cardiac arrest rhythms, including the reversible causes of cardiopulmonary arrest, are described in Chapter 9.

Considerations when using an AED

The AED pads are placed in the same position as manual defibrillators (Figure 8.1).

Sequence of actions for using an AED

The following guidance should be used for all AEDs, with or without a paediatric dose attenuating device:

1. Ensure safety of the child and rescuers/bystanders.

2. Start BLS (see Chapter 4).

3. Switch on the AED and attach self-adhesive pads. If more than one rescuer is present, BLS should be continued whilst the AED is attached.

4. Follow the AED prompts and ensure no-one touches the child while the rhythm is being analysed. (This is extremely important as artefact from chest compressions given during the analysis phase may be interpreted by the AED as VF, and the machine may charge and advise a shock).

5. If defibrillation is indicated, follow the AED prompts:
   - ensure no-one touches the child
   - press the shock delivery button as directed
   - continue as directed by the AED prompts.

6. If no shock is indicated:
   - resume BLS immediately
   - continue as directed by the AED prompts.

7. Continue resuscitation until:
   - help arrives and takes over management
   - the child starts to show signs of life
   - the rescuer becomes too exhausted to continue.

Note: do not switch off the AED whilst CPR is continued.

Considerations when undertaking synchronised DC cardioversion

Cardioversion is the first line of treatment for children and infants presenting with decompensated circulatory failure due to supraventricular tachycardia (SVT) or ventricular tachycardia with a pulse (VT). The delivery of the shock is synchronised with the R wave of the ECG to minimise the risk of inducing VF.

> Expert help must be sought if cardioversion is required.

The application of the pads and the safety precautions are the same as for asynchronous defibrillation, but there are some additional considerations. These include:

- Sedation/anaesthesia needs to be administered (if the child is conscious) before synchronised cardioversion is performed.
- Synchronisation mode on the defibrillator must be activated, and on some machines, it may need to be re-selected if repeat shock(s) are required.
- Increase the ECG gain to ensure the defibrillator identified all the R waves on the child's ECG.
- Energy levels for synchronised cardioversion are lower than for asynchronous defibrillation. The initial dose is 1 J kg⁻¹, although this may be increased to 2 J kg⁻¹ if the arrhythmia persists.
- ECG electrodes, in addition to pads, are needed for some defibrillators to operate in synchronised mode.
- Delays in shock delivery can occur between the operator depressing the delivery button and the actual shock being delivered. This is because the machine will only deliver the shock when it identifies an R wave. In practice, it means that the operator must keep the shock delivery button depressed until this occurs.

Following cardioversion, some defibrillators may remain in the synchronised mode, which is a potential risk; a defibrillator left in synchronised mode will not be immediately ready to deliver a shock to treat a VF/pVT cardiorespiratory arrest. Therefore, always leave the defibrillator in the non-synchronised mode.

08: Summary learning

For the patient in VF/pVT, early defibrillation is the only effective means of restoring a spontaneous circulation.

When using a defibrillator, minimise interruptions in chest compressions to reduce no-flow times.

Good communication and teamwork is essential to optimise outcome and overall safety.

Use an AED if you are not confident in rhythm recognition or manual defibrillation.

My key take-home messages from this chapter are:

Further reading

Atkinson E, Mikysa B et al. Specificity and sensitivity of automated external defibrillator rhythm analysis in infants and children. Ann Emerg Med 2003;42: 185-96

Benson D, Jr., Smith W, Dunnigan A, Sterba R, Gallagher J. Mechanisms of regular wide QRS tachycardia in infants and children. Am J Cardiol 1982;49:1778-88.

Berg RA, Chapman FW et al. Attenuated adult biphasic shocks compared with weight-based monophasic shocks in a swine model of prolonged pediatric ventricular fibrillation. Resuscitation 2004; 61: 189-197.

Berg RA, Samson RA et al. Better outcome after pediatric defibrillation dosage than adult dosage in a swine model of pediatric ventricular fibrillation. J Am Coll Cardiol 2005;45: 786-9.

Clark CB, Zhang Y et al. Pediatric transthoracic defibrillation: biphasic versus monophasic waveforms in an experimental model. Resuscitation 2001;51: 159-63.

Edelson DP, Abella BS, Kramer-Johansen J, et al. Effects of compression depth and pre-shock pauses predict defibrillation failure during cardiac arrest. Resuscitation 2006;71:137-45.

Eftestol T, Sunde K, Steen PA. Effects of interrupting precordial compressions on the calculated probability of defibrillation success during out-of-hospital cardiac arrest. Circulation 2002;105:2270-3.

Faddy SC, Powell J et al. Biphasic and monophasic shocks for transthoracic defibrillation: A meta analysis of randomised controlled trials. Resuscitation 2003;8: 9-16.

Jorgenson D, Morgan C, Snyder D et al. Energy attenuator for pediatric application of an automated external defibrillator. Crit Care Med 2002;30:S145-7.

Meaney P, Nadkarni V et al. Effect of defibrillation dose during in-hospital pediatric cardiac arrest. Pediatrics 2011;127(1):e16-23.

Rodriguez-Nunez A, Lopez-Herce J. Shockable rhythms and defibrillation during in-hospital pediatric cardiac arrest. Resuscitation 2014;85:387-91.

Rossano JQ, Schiff L, Kenney MA, Atkins DL. Survival is not correlated with defibrillation dosing in pediatric out-of-hospital ventricular fibrillation. Circulation 2003;108: IV-320-321.

Seeram N, Wren C. Supraventricular tachycardia in infants: response to initial treatment. Arch Dis Child 1990;65:127-9.

Samson R, Berg R et al. Use of automated external defibrillators for children: an update. An advisory statement from the Pediatric Advanced Life Support Task Force, International Liaison Committee on Resuscitation. Resuscitation 2003;57: 237-43.

Schneider T, Martens PR et al. Multicenter, randomised, controlled trial of 150 J biphasic shocks compared with 200- to 360 J monophasic shocks in the resuscitation of out-of-hospital cardiac arrest victims. Circulation 2000;102: 1780-1787.

Tibbals J, Carter B et al. External and internal biphasic direct current shock doses for pediatric VF and pulseless VT. Pediatric Crit Care Med 2011;12:14-20.

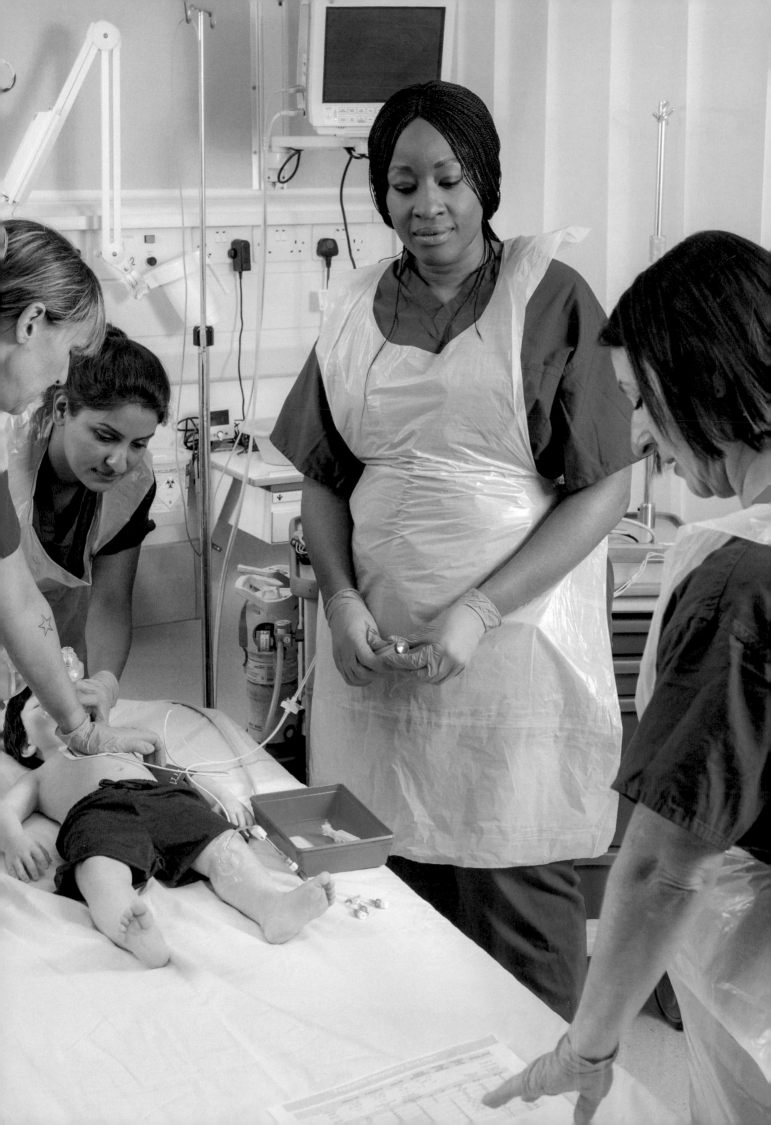

Management of cardiorespiratory arrest

Resuscitation process

Resuscitation is a continuous process from basic life support to advanced life support, with high-quality BLS providing the most important foundation for successful resuscitation. BLS must be continued until the return of a spontaneous circulation (ROSC), even when experienced help arrives (e.g. EMS, resuscitation teams, clinical emergency teams).

It is important that the on-call clinical emergency team/resuscitation team prepare for this event at the changeover of staff and team huddles (Chapter 11).

Throughout this chapter, all references to 'resuscitation teams' or 'rapid response teams' will be referred to as 'clinical emergency teams'.

All clinical staff within a healthcare facility should be able to:

*   immediately recognise cardiorespiratory arrest
*   start appropriate resuscitation (BLS with available adjuncts)
*   summon the clinical emergency team using the standard telephone number (2222 in-hospital) and/or EMS (via national 999 system).

The exact sequence of actions will be dependent on several factors, including:

*   location of the event (clinical or non-clinical area)
*   number of first responders
*   skills of first responders
*   availability of resuscitation equipment
*   local policies.

> High-quality BLS provides the most important foundation for successful resuscitation

Preventing cardiorespiratory arrest

If a child is seriously ill on a ward, it is likely that they will have been deteriorating over a period of time. Measures must be put in place to ensure any critically ill child is identified and transferred to a safe area with early admission to ICU/HDU where appropriate, the aim is to ensure the child is in the right bed at the right time. Many wards now employ early warning scoring (EWS) systems based on physiological parameters to help identify seriously ill children. Evidence from a large randomised trial indicated that whilst the implementation of an EWS system does not affect mortality, it can help improve recognition of the physiologically unstable child, reducing the number of critical incidents associated with deterioration on the wards. So, whilst early warning scores are useful as part of the overall clinical response system, there must also be a focus on improving healthcare providers' ability to recognise and intervene for patients with deteriorating illness. Monitored physiological parameters are particularly useful in looking at trends that can provide more useful information than a single elevated EWS score. It is always important to note any parental or nurse concern. All findings need to be escalated early, and appropriate management strategies are initiated to try and prevent cardiorespiratory arrest from occurring.

Summoning senior clinical support such as clinical emergency teams may reduce the risk of respiratory and/or cardiac arrest in hospitalised children and infants. The causes of the majority of cardiorespiratory arrests in children and infants arise from decompensated respiratory or circulatory failure causing hypoxia. Secondary cardiorespiratory arrests have a poor outcome, and hence the identification of the seriously ill or injured child is an absolute priority. Any unwell child should be assessed using the A–E assessment process and findings communicated to ensure the child is in a safe setting. When preventative measures and systems for early escalation for expert support are in place, a paediatric cardiorespiratory arrest outside of HDU, ITU or ED is thankfully a rare event.

Cardiorespiratory arrest in a clinical area

When a child does suffer a cardiorespiratory arrest in a clinical area, staff should be able to promptly initiate BLS and put out a 2222 call to summon the clinical emergency team. Appropriate resuscitation equipment and trained staff should be readily available.

Cardiorespiratory arrest in a non-clinical area

There may be occasions when a child suffers a cardiorespiratory arrest in a non-clinical area (e.g. corridors, car park, play area). In these areas, equipment or trained staff may not be readily available, and these children may have a more prolonged period of BLS before help arrives.

In-hospital cardiorespiratory arrest (IHCA)

The guidance in the first section of this chapter is primarily aimed at healthcare professionals who may be initial responders in a clinical emergency situation and have rapid access to resuscitation equipment. The guidance in the second section of this chapter is primarily aimed at the team providing experienced help, including guidance for the team leader.

Number of first responders

A single rescuer must not leave the collapsed child but should start appropriate resuscitation (e.g. BLS or BLS with BMV) and ensure that further help is summoned.

Within a clinical area, there are usually more staff nearby who can be alerted, either by the first responder shouting for help and/or using an emergency call button system. As soon as a second rescuer arrives, they should be sent to summon further assistance in line with local policy (i.e. activate the clinical emergency team via a 2222 call). On their return (or on the arrival of other staff), simultaneous interventions can be undertaken, according to the skills of the available staff.

Skills of first responders

Healthcare providers should be able to recognise cardiorespiratory arrest, shout for help and start resuscitation to the level to which they have been trained. The decay in resuscitation skills after training is well documented, with skills retention probably lasting about three months. Recent studies indicate that short, targeted refresher training for staff looking after the sicker patients at their bedsides may be beneficial, so-called 'just in time' training.

Staff will have been trained to different levels according to local policies; some may only undertake BLS, whilst others would be expected to undertake additional techniques to manage airway, breathing and circulation. The initial priority for first responders in paediatric cardiorespiratory arrest should be to ensure effective ventilation and oxygenation with good quality chest compressions. As more experienced help arrives, other interventions can be undertaken.

Figure 9.1   Team member positions to ensure 360° access to the patient

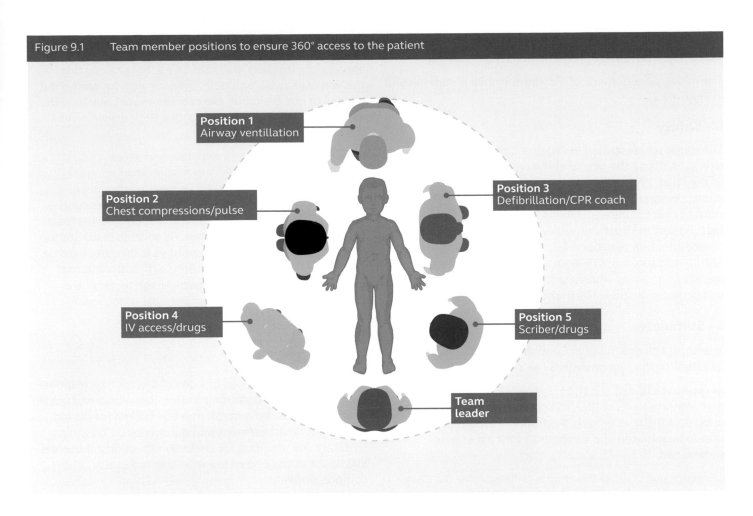

Availability of resuscitation equipment

All clinical areas where children are likely to be cared for should be equipped with resuscitation equipment to help manage a clinical emergency. The staff in each area should have responsibility for maintenance and regular checking of this clinical emergency equipment, as this will facilitate their familiarity with it. Standardised resuscitation equipment hospital-wide enables the clinical emergency teams to know what equipment is readily available to them when called to deal with a child in any area. Equipment capable of delivering CPR feedback for rescuers will improve the quality of CPR delivered and is strongly recommended.

Quality standards

Healthcare organisations have an obligation to provide a high-quality resuscitation service and to ensure that staff are trained and updated regularly and with appropriate frequency to a level of proficiency appropriate to each individual's expected role. The Resuscitation Council UK 'Quality Standards for Cardiopulmonary Resuscitation Practice and Training' provide further detailed information.

Hospitals should have policies regarding the composition of, and calling criteria for their clinical emergency teams. In some hospitals there might be more than one emergency team (dictated by the geographical layout or the clinical specialities of the hospital), or there may be different types of team (e.g. a cardiac arrest team and a medical emergency team). Staff must be aware of their local systems and trained to act accordingly.

As clinical emergency teams members will differ daily, it is invaluable that team huddle/meet at the beginning of each shift. These 'huddles' enable the team members to introduce themselves to each other, discuss each team member's skills, assign roles, and identify those patients with a high risk of deterioration across the hospital. These 'huddles' can improve teamwork, particularly communication in a subsequent emergency scenario. Clinical emergency teams will operate more efficiently if skills can be practiced and refreshed regularly by undertaking 'mock' emergency calls; these will enable team members to refresh ALS knowledge and practice team "choreography" which will improve performance (Figure 9.1).

The sequence of actions in cardiopulmonary resuscitation (CPR)

The initial management of a collapsed child is summarised in Figure 9.2.

S – Safety

The approach described in Chapter 4 should be followed to ensure firstly the safety of the rescuers and then that of the child. Whilst the risk of contracting an infection is low, personal protective measures should be used as soon as practicable (e.g. gloves, aprons, eye protection, face masks). In situations where the child may have a severe infection (e.g. open TB, COVID-19, Swine flu or SARS), rescuers must be equipped with full protective measures. In areas where such children may be treated, this equipment should be immediately available.

S– Stimulate

The approach described in Chapter 4 should be followed to establish the responsiveness of an unconscious child.

Responsive child: If the child responds (i.e. they demonstrate signs of life), the child should be assessed using an ABCDE approach. Appropriate interventions should be initiated and further relevant assistance summoned.

Unresponsive child: If the child is unresponsive (i.e. they do not demonstrate signs of life), start BLS immediately whilst simultaneously shouting for more assistance.

S – Shout for help

The single-rescuer must not leave the child but shout loudly for help and start BLS, using basic airway adjuncts and BMV if they are immediately available and activating a bedside emergency call button system if this is available.

If there is a second rescuer available, they should be sent to summon more assistance and return to help with the resuscitation attempt.

If resuscitation equipment is nearby, they should bring this to the bedside, but this must not delay calling the clinical emergency team.

Airway

The airway should be opened as described in Chapters 3 and 4. If suction is available, it may be necessary to use this to clear any secretions in the upper airway before proceeding to ventilation.

Breathing

The rescuer should perform a breathing check, as described in Chapter 4, for 10 seconds whilst looking for signs of life (responsiveness, coughing, spontaneous movements, and normal breathing).

If the child is not breathing or only gasping ineffectively, initial rescue breaths should be delivered by the most appropriate method available. In the hospital setting, this will usually be with a BMV device with supplemental oxygen (if not available, expired air rescue breaths with a barrier device may be used until a BMV device can be retrieved).

If there are two rescuers available and at least one is trained in the use of BMV, the rescuer managing the airway and delivering the rescue breaths should be positioned behind the child's head. A second rescuer should be positioned at the side of the child to perform chest compressions if indicated. As soon as resuscitation equipment is available, the emphasis is on ensuring that effective CPR is enhanced by BMV with supplemental oxygen. When using BMV, a two-person technique is advocated to provide an adequate seal of the mask.

Circulation

Assessment

The presence or absence of signs of life, such as response to stimuli, normal breathing (rather than abnormal gasps) or spontaneous movement, must be looked for during the breathing assessment and during rescue breathing to determine the need for chest compressions. If there is still doubt at the end of the rescue breaths, start chest compressions.

Feeling for a pulse is not a reliable way to determine if there is an effective or inadequate circulation, and palpation of the pulse is not the determinant of the need for chest compressions. Rescuers are no longer taught to feel for a pulse as part of assessing the need for chest compressions in BLS. If a healthcare provider still wishes to do a pulse check in an unresponsive child, they must be certain that one is present for them NOT to start CPR. In this situation, there are often other signs of life present.

High-quality chest compressions are extremely important to maximise the chances of successful CPR. The components are:

- correct compression rate: 100–120 min^{-1} for both infants and children
- correct depth: release all pressure on the chest between compressions to allow for complete chest recoil and avoid leaning on the chest at the end of a compression
- pauses in chest compressions should be planned and minimised so that 80% or more of the CPR cycle is comprised of chest compressions (this is also known as chest compression fraction)
- ventilations and compressions are then delivered in a 15:2 ratio until monitoring is attached to guide specific management.

Paediatric basic life support

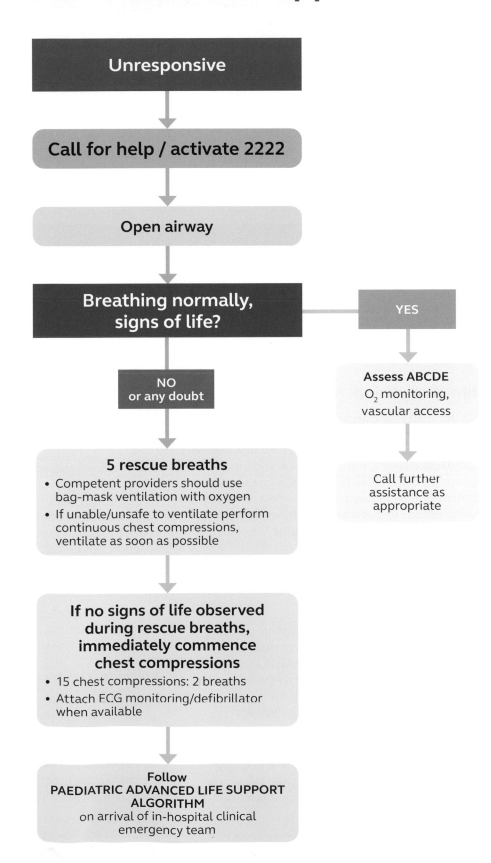

Figure 9.2   Initial resuscitation management

95

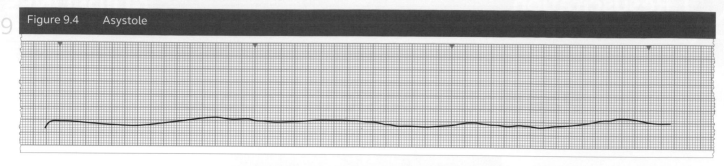

Figure 9.4   Asystole

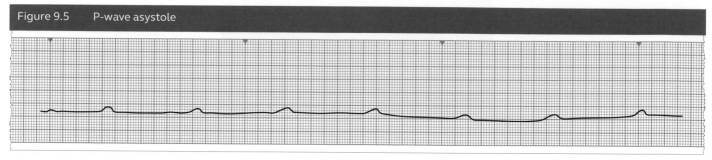

Figure 9.5   P-wave asystole

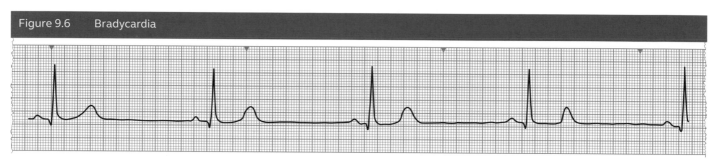

Figure 9.6   Bradycardia

Rhythm recognition

Establish the child's cardiac rhythm by attaching ECG monitoring (available on manual defibrillators) or defibrillator pads (preferably with a CPR feedback sensor). The priority is deciding whether the cardiac rhythm is shockable or non-shockable to determine the ongoing management of the cardiorespiratory arrest. Briefly pause chest compressions to allow for rhythm recognition on the monitor. If an AED is used, it will guide the rescuers through the sequence of actions.

Shockable or non-shockable cardiac rhythms

In children, the most common initial cardiorespiratory arrest rhythms are non-shockable (i.e. profound bradycardia, asystole or pulseless electrical activity (PEA). CPR should be started in children who become bradycardic (heart rate < 60 min⁻¹) with signs of inadequate perfusion despite adequate respiratory support and oxygenation.

The shockable cardiorespiratory arrest rhythms (i.e. ventricular fibrillation (VF) and pulseless ventricular tachycardia (pVT)) are less common. When these occur, it is often in a child with underlying cardiac disease (congenital or acquired).

The management of shockable and non-shockable cardiorespiratory arrest is outlined in Figure 9.3.

Non-shockable rhythms (asystole and PEA)

Asystole

This rhythm is characterised by the total absence of effective electrical and mechanical activity in the heart (Figure 9.4). It can be simulated by artefact (e.g. detached ECG leads/electrodes), so it is important to quickly check the equipment. In asystole, there is no ventricular function, but occasionally there is some atrial activity, which may be seen on the ECG as P waves (Figure 9.5). It is often preceded by severe bradycardia (Figure 9.6). The most common cause of bradycardia in a child is hypoxia, but hypotension, hypothermia or hypoglycaemia can depress normal cardiac activity and slow conduction through cardiac tissues.

Pulseless electrical activity (PEA)

This rhythm is defined as organised cardiac electrical activity in the absence of signs of life. Some of these children may have some myocardial contraction, but it is too weak and ineffective to produce a detectable pulse, blood pressure or signs of life. The ECG rhythm displayed is often a slow, broad complex one, although any variation of regular QRS complexes may be seen.

All the cardiorespiratory arrest rhythms may be due to an underlying reversible condition; identify and treat all reversible causes listed within the paediatric advanced life support algorithm (Figure 9.10, Table 9.1).

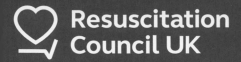

Paediatric advanced life support

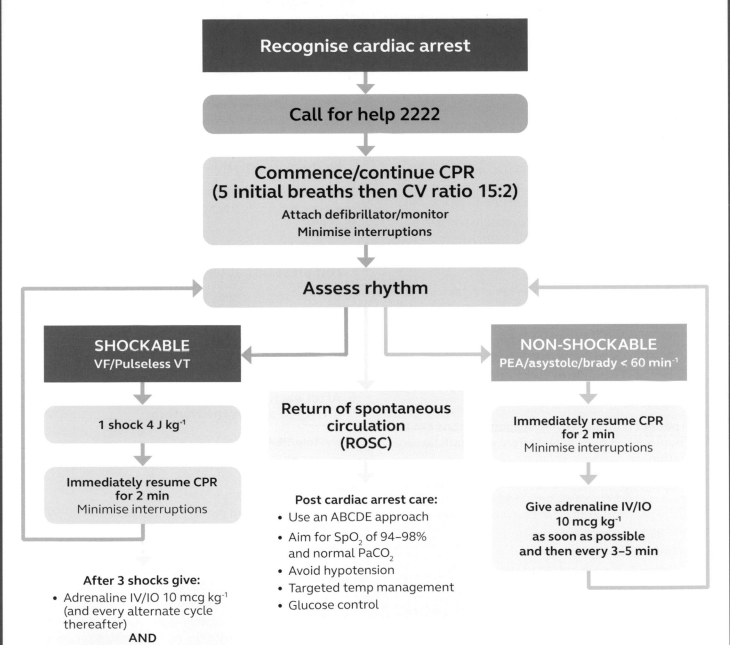

Recognise cardiac arrest

Call for help 2222

Commence/continue CPR
(5 initial breaths then CV ratio 15:2)
Attach defibrillator/monitor
Minimise interruptions

Assess rhythm

SHOCKABLE
VF/Pulseless VT

NON-SHOCKABLE
PEA/asystolc/brady < 60 min⁻¹

1 shock 4 J kg⁻¹

Return of spontaneous circulation (ROSC)

Immediately resume CPR for 2 min
Minimise interruptions

Immediately resume CPR for 2 min
Minimise interruptions

Give adrenaline IV/IO 10 mcg kg⁻¹
as soon as possible and then every 3–5 min

Post cardiac arrest care:
- Use an ABCDE approach
- Aim for SpO_2 of 94–98% and normal $PaCO_2$
- Avoid hypotension
- Targeted temp management
- Glucose control

After 3 shocks give:
- Adrenaline IV/IO 10 mcg kg⁻¹ (and every alternate cycle thereafter)
          AND
- Amiodarone IV/IO 5 mg kg⁻¹ (and repeat 5 mg kg⁻¹ once more only after 5th shock)

During CPR
- **Ensure high quality chest compressions are delivered:**
  – Correct rate, depth and full recoil
- Provide BMV with 100% oxygen (2 person approach)
- Provide continuous chest compressions when a tracheal tube is in place.
- Competent providers can consider an advanced airway and capnography, and ventilate at a rate (breaths minute⁻¹) of:

Infants: 25	1–8 years: 20	8–12 years: 15	> 12 years: 10–12

- Vascular access IV/IO
- Once started, give Adrenaline every 3-5 min
- Maximum single dose Adrenaline 1 mg
- Maximum single dose Amiodarone 300 mg

Identify and treat reversible causes
- Hypoxia
- Hypovolaemia
- Hyperkalaemia, hypercalcaemia, hypermagnesemia, hypoglycaemia
- Hypo-/hyperthermia
- Thrombosis – coronary or pulmonary
- Tension pneumothorax
- Tamponade – cardiac
- Toxic agents

Adjust algorithm in specific settings (e.g. special circumstances)

Figure 9.3   Paediatric advanced life support algorithm

Management of asystole and PEA

1. Perform CPR

- Continue to ventilate with high concentration oxygen. Provide ventilation initially by bag-mask ventilation (BMV), using high-concentration inspired oxygen 100% as soon as this is available. Do not titrate the concentration of inspired oxygen during CPR. To provide an adequate seal of the mask, a two-person technique is advocated.

- If ventilating with a bag-mask use a ratio of 15 chest compressions to 2 ventilations.

- Use a compression rate of 100–120 min^{-1}. Depth of compressions is one-third of the depth of the chest, approximately 4 cm in an infant and 5 cm in a child.

- When performing chest compressions, choose a team member who will be able to deliver them most effectively and use a rigid surface/backboard so that chest compressions are more effective

- If BMV can be successfully performed, then continue with this mode of ventilation. A team member with the necessary skills to safely intubate the child or infant should intubate the trachea only if this can be performed with minimal interruption to chest compressions. A supraglottic airway (SGA) can be used as an alternative until a competent provider can intubate.

If the patient is intubated, chest compressions can be continuous if this does not interfere with satisfactory ventilation.

Once the child's trachea has been intubated and effective continuous chest compressions underway, ventilation should be provided at the lower limit of the normal rate for their age:

- **Infants:** 25 breaths per min
- **Children 1–8 years old:** 20 breaths per min
- **Children 8–12 years old:** 15 breaths per min
- **Children over 12 years old:** 10–12 breaths per min.

Note: Once there is ROSC, the ventilation rate should be a normal physiological age-dependent respiratory rate which may then be adjusted to meet the goals of post-resuscitation care. Measure end-tidal carbon dioxide (end-tidal CO_2) to monitor ventilation and ensure correct TT placement.

2. Give adrenaline as soon as possible

For non-shockable rhythms, the first dose of adrenaline should be given as soon as possible; administer adrenaline 10 micrograms kg^{-1} (0.1 mL kg^{-1} of a 1:10 000 solution) IV/IO, preferably within 3 min of identification of cardiorespiratory arrest.

Once the first dose of adrenaline has been given, continue to administer adrenaline every 3–5 min (i.e. every other cycle) while maintaining effective chest compressions and ventilation without interruption.

3. Continue CPR, only pausing briefly every 2 min to check for rhythm changes

The aim is to maximise chest compressions time, and the chest compressions fraction should be equal to or greater than 80%.

4. Change the person performing chest compressions at least every 2 min

Watch for fatigue and/or suboptimal compressions and switch rescuers earlier if necessary.

5. Consider and correct reversible causes:

Consider the relevant 4 H's and 4 T's.

6. After each 2 min of uninterrupted CPR, pause briefly to assess the rhythm:

If asystole/PEA:

- Continue CPR using the non-shockable sequence.

If VF/pVT:

- Continue CPR and switch to the shockable (VF/pVT) side of the algorithm.

- If organised electrical activity is seen, check for signs of life and a pulse:
  - If there is ROSC, continue post-resuscitation care.
  - If there is no pulse (or a pulse rate of < 60 min^{-1}), and there are no other signs of life, continue CPR and continue with the non-shockable sequence above.

- Feeling for a pulse:
  - In an infant – feel for the brachial pulse on the inner aspect of the upper arm.
  - In a child aged over 1 year – feel for the carotid pulse in the neck.
  - For both infants and children, the femoral pulse in the groin (mid-way between the anterior superior iliac spine and the symphysis pubis) can also be used.

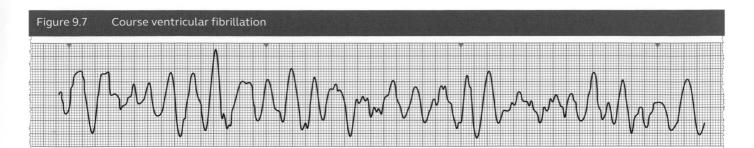

Figure 9.7   Course ventricular fibrillation

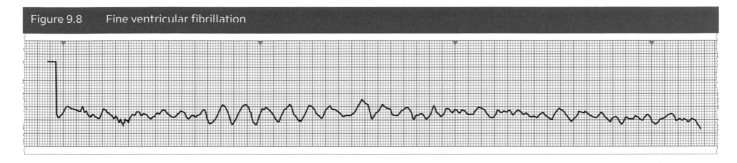

Figure 9.8   Fine ventricular fibrillation

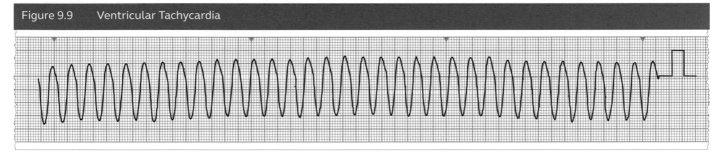

Figure 9.9   Ventricular Tachycardia

Shockable rhythms (VF and pVT)

Ventricular fibrillation

This rhythm shows rapid, chaotic, irregular waves of varying frequency and amplitude. VF is sometimes classified as 'coarse or fine' depending on the amplitude (height) of the complexes (Figures 9.7 and 9.8). As soon as identified, defibrillation should immediately be attempted (regardless of the ECG amplitude). If in doubt, consider the rhythm to be shockable. Shockable rhythms are less common in children but may occur as a secondary event and are more likely when there has been a witnessed and sudden collapse. It is seen more often in the intensive care unit and cardiac ward or in adolescents on the sporting field.

Pulseless ventricular tachycardia (pVT)

This rhythm is a broad complex tachycardia (Figure 9.9). It is rare in children and is managed in the same way as VF (i.e. defibrillation).

Management of VF/pVT

1. **Continue CPR until a defibrillator is available.**

2. **Apply defibrillation pads** (self-adhesive pads are standard) in the antero-lateral or antero-posterior position, if not yet in place.

3. **Defibrillate** (as soon as possible):

   • Charge the defibrillator while another rescuer continues chest compressions, all other rescuers must stand clear during this time.

   • Once the defibrillator is charged, pause the chest compressions, quickly ensure that all rescuers are clear of the patient and then deliver the shock. Minimise the delay between stopping chest compressions and delivery of the shock (< 5 seconds).

   • Deliver 1 shock of 4 J kg⁻¹ if using a manual defibrillator. It seems reasonable not to use doses above those suggested for adults.

   • If using an AED for a child of less than 8 years, if an attenuator is available, deliver a paediatric attenuated adult shock energy (50–75 J). If an attenuator is not available, use a standard AED which will deliver adult shock energy doses.

   • If using an AED for a child over 8 years, use the adult shock energy.

4. **Resume CPR:**
   - Without reassessing the rhythm or feeling for a pulse, resume CPR immediately, starting with chest compressions.
   - Good quality CPR can be maximised if a feedback device is used.

5. **Continue CPR for 2 min, then pause briefly to check the monitor:**
   - If still VF/pVT, give a second shock (with the same energy level 4 J kg^{-1}) and strategy for delivery as the first shock).

6. **Resume CPR:**
   - Without reassessing the rhythm or feeling for a pulse, resume CPR immediately, starting with chest compressions.

7. **Continue CPR for 2 min, then pause briefly to check the monitor**

8. **If still VF/pVT, deliver a third shock** (with the same energy level 4 J kg^{-1} and strategy for delivery as the previous shock).

9. **Resume CPR:**
   - Without reassessing the rhythm or feeling for a pulse, resume CPR immediately, starting with chest compressions.
   - With chest compressions ongoing, give adrenaline 10 micrograms kg^{-1} (0.1 mL kg^{-1} of 1:10 000 solution) and amiodarone 5 mg kg^{-1} after the third shock.
   - Repeat adrenaline 10 micrograms kg^{-1} (0.1 mL kg^{-1} of 1:10 000 solution) every alternate cycle (every 3–5 min) until ROSC.
   - Repeat amiodarone 5 mg kg^{-1} one further time after the fifth shock if still in a shockable rhythm.

10. **Continue delivering shocks every 2 min**, continuing compressions during charging of the defibrillator and minimising the breaks in chest compressions as much as possible.
    - Change the person performing chest compressions at least every 2 min, Watch for fatigue and/or suboptimal compressions and switch rescuers earlier if necessary.
    - Consider and correct reversible causes (4 H's and 4 T's)
    - After each 2 min of uninterrupted CPR, pause briefly to assess the rhythm.

    If still VF/pVT:
    - Continue CPR with the shockable (VF/pVT) sequence.

If asystole/PEA:
- Continue CPR and switch to the non-shockable (asystole or PEA) sequence.

If organised electrical activity is seen, check for signs of life and a pulse:
- If there is ROSC, continue post-resuscitation care.
- If there is no pulse (or a pulse rate of < 60 min^{-1}), and there are no other signs of life, continue CPR as for the non-shockable sequence.

11. **If defibrillation was successful but VF/pVT recurs,** resume the CPR sequence and defibrillate. Give an amiodarone bolus (unless two doses have already been administered) and start a continuous infusion of the drug.

12. **CPR should be continued unless:**
    - An organised perfusing rhythm is recognised and confirmed by a clinical assessment indicating signs of life (ROSC).
    - There are criteria for withdrawing resuscitation.

13. **After the event, debriefing of the team** should be conducted to express any concerns and to allow the team to reflect on their clinical practice in a supportive environment (this has been shown to improve practice).

Important notes

- Good team planning before each action will minimise hands-off time and improve the quality of CPR.
- Studies show that visual assessment of depth of compressions is inaccurate; therefore, where possible, feedback devices may be utilised. When correct guidelines are followed, chest compressions depth and rate achieved, the chances of survival are markedly improved.
- The interval between stopping chest compressions and delivering a shock must be minimal; longer interruptions reduce the likelihood of a shock restoring a perfusing rhythm.
- Chest compressions are resumed immediately after a shock without reassessing the rhythm or feeling for a pulse because, even if the defibrillation attempt is successful in restoring a rhythm, it is unlikely that the heart will immediately pump effectively. Giving further chest compressions does not increase the chance of VF recurring.
- If an organised rhythm is observed during a 2 min cycle of CPR, do not interrupt chest compressions to palpate a pulse unless the patient shows signs of life demonstrating the return of spontaneous circulation (ROSC).

Airway and ventilation

The vast majority of children can be adequately ventilated with BMV in the initial stages of resuscitation. It is often better to continue with this strategy until ROSC, rather than attempt tracheal intubation and temporarily interrupt chest compressions and oxygenation during laryngoscopy.

If BMV is unsuccessful and a team member with the necessary skills to safely intubate the child or infant is not yet present, a suitably trained provider may use a supraglottic airway (SGA) as an alternative.

A tracheal tube (TT) provides the most reliable airway. As soon as the airway is secured with a TT, chest compressions should be performed continuously unless this compromises the delivery of adequate tidal volumes.

If laryngoscopy is to be performed during CPR, it should be attempted without interruption of chest compressions, although there may need to be a brief pause as the TT is passed through the vocal cords.

End-tidal CO_2 should be continuously monitored once a TT or SGA is in place:

- The absence of exhaled CO_2 during CPR should prompt providers to check tracheal tube placement, remember, **'no trace, wrong place'**.

- Once there is a sustained return of spontaneous circulation (ROSC), titrate the oxygen to an SpO_2 of 94–98%. In children and infants who do not regain consciousness or for other clinical indications, an advanced airway may be required. Team members with the necessary skills to insert an advanced airway will be required (drugs may be needed at this point to assist).

- For children or infants already on a mechanical ventilator at the time of cardiac arrest, either continue to ventilate with the ventilator or disconnect and ventilate by means of a self-inflating bag. In the latter case, ensure that the ventilator is in a volume-controlled mode, that triggers and limits are disabled, and ventilation rate, tidal volume and the fraction of inspired oxygen (FiO_2) are appropriate for CPR. Ventilator dysfunction can itself be a cause of cardiorespiratory arrest.

History and reversible causes

Obtaining relevant information about the child's underlying medical condition and any pre-disposing events can be useful in determining likely causes of and potential outcomes from the cardiorespiratory arrest. The early identification and proper treatment of any reversible causes during CPR is a priority for all ALS providers (Table 9.1, Figure 9.10).

The four H's and 4 T's

Use the mnemonic '4 H's and 4 T's' to remember what to actively look for:

- Hypoxia
- Hypovolemia
- Hypo- or hyperkalaemia / -calcaemia / -magnesaemia and hypoglycaemia
- Hypo- or hyperthermia
- Tension pneumothorax
- Tamponade
- Thrombosis (Cardiac or pulmonary)
- Toxic agents.

Table 9.1   Reversible causes of cardiorespiratory arrest

Consider	Identification:	Treatment
Hypoxia	History/clinical exam +/-oxygen saturation (if trace picked up)	Ventilation with 100% FiO_2
Hypovolaemia	History +/- POCUS*	Fluid bolus 10 mL kg⁻¹ isotonic crystalloid; blood products (major haemorrhage)
Hyper/hypokalaemia	History + blood gas analysis	Correction/reduction of metabolic derangement
Hypothermia/ Hyperthermia	History + core temperature	External (e.g. blanket), internal (e.g. cold/warm fluids, extracorporeal circuit) techniques
Thromboembolism	History +/- POCUS* (e.g. dilated right ventricle)	IV thrombolysis
Tension pneumothorax	Examine symmetrical air entry +/- POCUS*	Needle thoracocentesis/ thoracostomy (trauma)
Tamponade (cardiac)	History +/- POCUS * (e.g. pericardial fluid collection).	Needle pericardiocentesis/ thoracotomy (trauma)
Toxic	History / ECG	Specific toxic treatment (e.g. sodium bicarbonate for tricyclic drug poisoning)
*POCUS: point of care ultrasound – if competent operator available.		

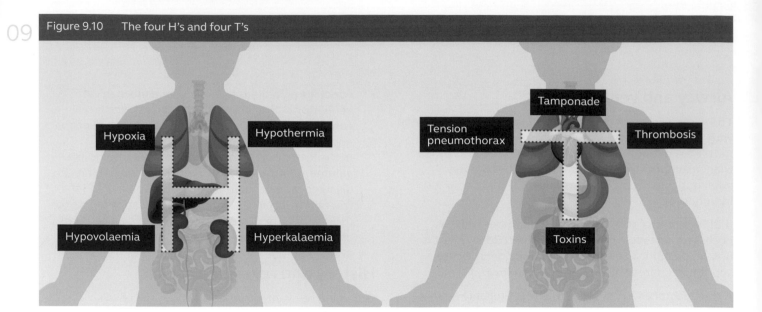

Figure 9.10   The four H's and four T's

Unless otherwise specified, the specific treatment for each of these causes is the same in cardiorespiratory arrest as in acute life-threatening disease.

Hypoxia

This is a frequent cause of paediatric cardiorespiratory arrest. The risks of it occurring, or persisting, during resuscitation should be minimised by ensuring effective ventilation with 100% oxygen. It is essential to ensure that there is adequate bilateral chest movement.

Hypovolaemia

Loss of circulating volume can often result in cardiorespiratory arrest. When a child shows signs of circulatory failure, controlled volume administration is indicated. Hypovolaemia may be due to many different causes (e.g. haemorrhage from trauma, diarrhoea and vomiting, anaphylaxis, severe sepsis), and these need to be identified and treated appropriately. If a clinical presentation or history suggests hypovolaemia, start rapid circulatory volume replacement with an initial bolus of isotonic balanced crystalloid or 0.9% sodium chloride; volume and frequency of bolus is discussed in Chapter 6.

Hypo/hyperkalaemia, metabolic causes

Electrolyte and metabolic disorders may be suggested by the child's medical history and/or biochemical tests.

Specific treatment should be given to correct these problems. An estimation of blood glucose level should be obtained early as both hypo- and hyperglycaemia are common and associated with increased morbidity and mortality.

Hypothermia and Hyperthermia

Low body temperature may be an unlikely problem in hospitalised children, but it should always be considered, particularly in small or premature infants or in children being managed in the emergency department.
A low-reading thermometer should be used to record a core temperature when hypothermia is considered a possibility. If the child's temperature is > 34°C they should not be actively rewarmed.

Tension pneumothorax

Signs of tension pneumothorax (e.g. decreased chest movement and air entry, hyperresonance on the affected side, tracheal deviation away from the affected side) should be sought, particularly in children who have suffered trauma, following thoracic surgery or jugular or subclavian vein central line insertion. If a tension pneumothorax is thought to be present, rapid needle decompression is required (or thoracostomy in trauma settings), followed by chest drain insertion.

Tamponade (cardiac)

This is not a common cause of cardiorespiratory arrest in children but may occur following cardiothoracic surgery, penetrating chest trauma or some viral illnesses. It can be difficult to diagnose as typical signs (e.g. distended neck veins and hypovolaemia) are often masked by the cardiorespiratory arrest. If there is a strong history, thoracotomy or needle pericardiocentesis is indicated.

Toxins

In the absence of a confirmed history, accidental or deliberate poisoning with toxins (therapeutic or toxic substances (e.g. digoxin toxicity, tricyclic antidepressant overdose)) may only be discovered after laboratory analysis. Appropriate antidotes should be administered as soon as possible when indicated and available (e.g. sodium bicarbonate in tricyclic poisonings); seek advice from a poisons centre for up-to-date guidance for severe or uncommon poisonings. However, the management of these children is frequently based on measures to support their vital organs. Remember to also check the child's drug chart.

Thrombosis (coronary or pulmonary)

It is unusual for children to suffer from thromboembolic complications, but they can occur. If suspected, appropriate thrombolysis would be needed (e.g. alteplase as per local guidelines).

Stopping resuscitation

Resuscitation efforts are less likely to be successful in achieving ROSC if there have been no signs of cardiac output, despite at least 30 min of continuous, good quality CPR in children. However, occasionally good quality survival has been reported for longer durations of CPR, so the circumstances of the cardiorespiratory arrest and the presenting rhythm must all be taken into consideration when making the decision to stop resuscitation. CPR is more often successful in children < 1 year of age and in those presenting with VF or pVT.

It would be appropriate to prolong resuscitation attempts in children with the following conditions:

- hypothermia
- poisoning
- persistent VF/pVT
- thrombolysis.

The resuscitation team may also consider that specific circumstances (e.g. awaiting the arrival of family members) make it appropriate to maintain resuscitation efforts.

After the event, debriefing of the event should be conducted to express any concerns and to allow the team to reflect on their clinical practice in a supportive environment.

A record of the event should be written in real-time. This should be completed by a senior member of the resuscitation team and allocated by the team leader. The scribe's notes should then be added if necessary and countersigned by all team members who took an active part in the event (e.g. anaesthetist, ICU medic, nurses etc.).

Presence of parents/guardians during resuscitation

The opportunity to be present during at least part of the resuscitation of their child should be offered to parents/guardians. Evidence suggests that most parents want to be present during a resuscitation attempt, and this can aid with their grieving process (less anxiety and depression was noted when assessed several months later). Reports show that being at the side of the child or infant is comforting to the parents or careers and helps them gain a realistic view of attempted resuscitation and death.

The following points (which apply whether the parent/guardian is actually in the room besides their child or elsewhere in the ward/department) should be considered:

- A specific member of staff should be delegated to remain with them throughout to offer empathetic but realistic support. They can also ensure the parents/guardians do not distract the resuscitation team.
- If necessary, an appropriate interpreter must be present to facilitate the accuracy of communication between parents/guardians and the resuscitation team leader.
- When appropriate, physical contact with their child during the event should be allowed.
- Time to say 'goodbye' (in unsuccessful resuscitation attempts) should be encouraged.
- The resuscitation team leader decides when to stop resuscitation efforts and not the parents/guardians.
- Appropriate referrals and counselling should be organised for the parents/guardians to ensure they receive adequate support.

09: Summary learning

The optimal management of in-hospital cardiorespiratory arrest is always based on the rapid initiation of effective ventilation, oxygenation and good quality chest compressions.

The paediatric advanced life support algorithm provides a framework for cardiorespiratory arrest management with an emphasis on providing high-quality CPR with minimal interruptions in chest compressions delivery.

Asystole and PEA are non-shockable arrhythmias, and their management is based on effective CPR, adrenaline administration and treatment of reversible causes.

VF and pVT are shockable arrhythmias, and their management is based on effective CPR, early defibrillation and treatment of reversible causes.

The parents/guardians should be supported and, ideally, be present during the resuscitation of their child.

My key take-home messages from this chapter are:

Further reading

Eppich WJ, Brannen M, Hunt EA: Team training: Implications for emergency and critical care pediatrics. Curr Opin Pediatr 2008;20:255-260.

Hanson CC, Randolph GD, Erickson JA, Mayer CM, et al. A reduction in cardiac arrests and duration of clinical instability after implementation of a paediatric rapid response system. Postgrad Med J 2010;86:314-318.

TIMMIS, V. 2020. Should family members be present at resuscitation? Arch Dis Child, 105, 506-508.

WALKER, W. & GAVIN, C. 2019. Family presence during resuscitation: A narrative review of the practices and views of critical care nurses. Intensive Crit Care Nurs, 53, 15-22.

Oczkowski SJ, Mazzetti, I, Cupido C, Fox-Robichaud AE; 2015. Canadian Critical care Society. Family presence during resuscitation. A CanadianCritical Care Society. position paper. Can Respir J, 4: 201 – 5

Thomas EJ, Williams AL, Reichman EF, Lasky RE, et al. Team training in the neonatal resuscitation program for interns: Teamwork and quality of resuscitations. Pediatrics 2010;125:539-546.

Weinstock P, Halamek LP: Teamwork during resuscitation. Pediatr Clin North Am 2008;55:1011-1024, xi-xii.

Early warning scores in Paediatrics: an overview. SM Chapman, IK Maconochie Archives of disease in childhood 104 (4), 395-399,2019

Effect of a Paediatric Early Warning System on All-Cause Mortality in Pediatric Patients: The EPOCH Randomised Clinical Trial. Christopher S Parshuram et al JAMA 2018

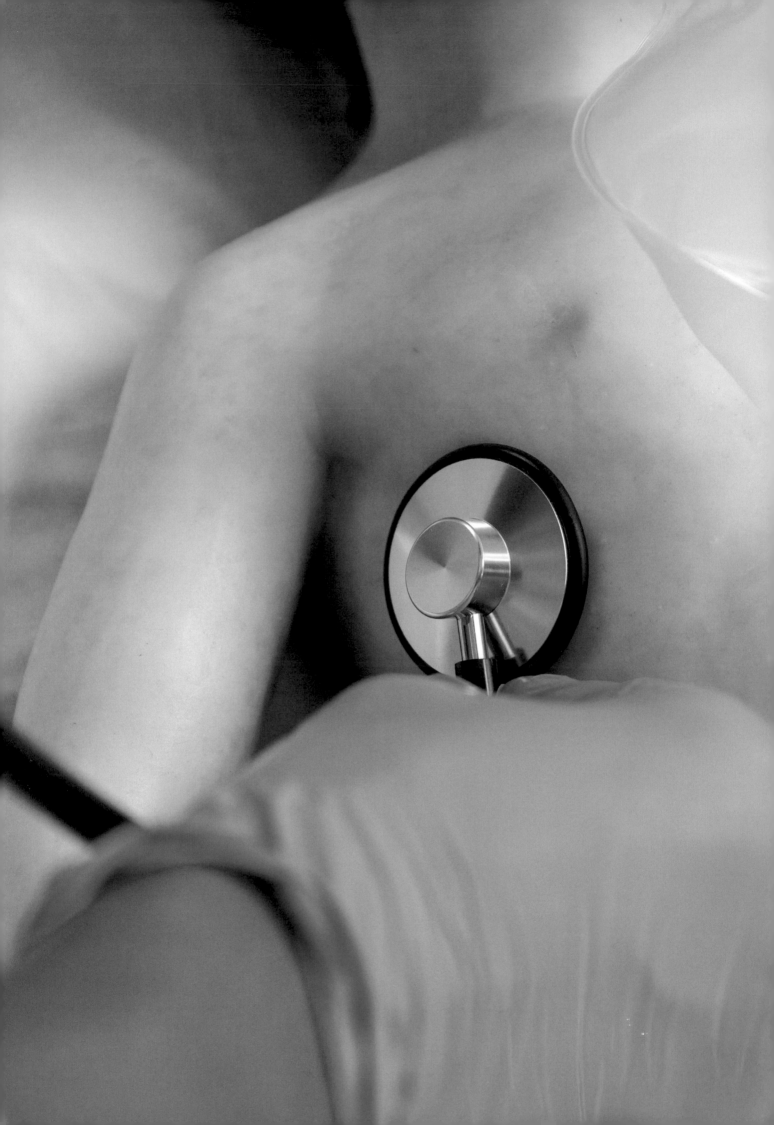

Post-resuscitation care, stabilisation and transfer

10

Continued resuscitation

Cardiorespiratory arrest represents the most severe shock state during which delivery of oxygen and metabolic substrates to tissues is abruptly halted. Cardiopulmonary resuscitation (CPR) only partially reverses this process, achieving cardiac output and systemic oxygen delivery that is much less than normal.

The aim of post-resuscitation care is to restore oxygenation and perfusion to the vital organs as rapidly as possible to minimise the primary injury. For children who have had a cardiorespiratory arrest, the initial step is the restoration of spontaneous circulation (ROSC), but this is only the first step in the continuous process of resuscitation management.

A significant percentage of resuscitated children ultimately die or survive with serious neurological sequelae, so good post-resuscitation care is required to maintain organ perfusion and prevent secondary organ injury whenever possible.

Secondary organ damage includes:

- hypoxic-ischaemic brain injury
- ischaemic myocardial damage
- hypoxic pulmonary damage
- acute kidney injury
- coagulopathy
- ischaemic hepatitis
- acute gastrointestinal lesions.

The ABCDE approach must be followed in the immediate post-resuscitation phase as it focuses management priorities. However, the ongoing care of the child requires the expertise of many healthcare professionals and is best delivered in a paediatric intensive care unit (PICU). This may require a specialist team to perform the critical care transfer.

> Good post-resuscitation care is required to maintain organ perfusion and prevent secondary organ injury whenever possible

A B Stabilisation of airway and breathing

The aim of respiratory management is to maintain adequate oxygenation and ventilation, avoiding hypoxia, hyperoxia, hypocapnia and hypercapnia, which may worsen the child's prognosis.

If the child (or infant) has been resuscitated using BMV, a decision needs to be made whether they will need ongoing ventilation and placement of a tracheal tube. Factors that may affect this decision include:

- conscious level (AVPU) at level P or less means that there may be reduced or absent protective airway reflexes
- requirement for the safe transfer to a PICU
- lung pathology resulting in a need for respiratory support.

BMV causes gastric distention which will impede ventilation and may cause vomiting. A gastric tube is usually required to deflate the stomach if it has become distended following BMV.

Children and infants who remain intubated and ventilated will need sedation and analgesia in most cases.

Following intubation, the most common post-resuscitation airway/breathing complications can be identified by considering the acronym DOPES (Table 10.1).

Table 10.1   Possible airway and breathing complications following tracheal intubation

D	Displacement of the tracheal tube (e.g. oesophagus, right main bronchus)
O	Obstruction of artificial airway (accumulated secretions (e.g. bronchiolitis), kinking of the tracheal tube)
P	Pneumothorax (from excessive BMV pressure, rib fractures)
E	Equipment failure (e.g. disconnected oxygen supply)
S	Stomach distension (following expired air or bag-mask ventilation)

Vital signs, such as heart rate, blood pressure, SpO_2 and end-tidal CO_2, blood glucose and temperature must be monitored post-resuscitation; blood gases can be used to further aid management.

Although 100% oxygen is used for resuscitation, prolonged administration of high oxygen concentrations can result in pulmonary and cerebral toxicity. Once the child is stable, titrate oxygen to achieve normoxaemia or, if arterial blood gas is not available, maintain SpO_2 in the range of 94–98%.

Exceptions are for children who have suffered smoke inhalation (carbon monoxide or cyanide poisoning) or have severe anaemia when a high FiO_2 should be maintained as dissolved O_2 helps in oxygen transport in these circumstances.

End-tidal CO_2 monitoring is mandatory. This will confirm the correct placement of a tracheal tube, allow continuous CO_2 monitoring during transport and support the optimisation of ventilation to maintain normocapnia. A chest X-ray should be obtained to check the position of the tracheal tube, gastric tube and central line if inserted in the neck. The tracheal tube may need to be re-positioned so that it is in an optimal position. You should also look for any lung pathology and check for any rib fractures (very rare in children) (Figure 10.1).

Provide a normal ventilatory rate and volume for the child's age to achieve a normal $PaCO_2$. Avoid both hypocapnia and hypercapnia. In a few children, the usual values for $PaCO_2$ and PaO_2 may deviate from the population normal values for age (e.g. in children with chronic lung disease or congenital heart conditions); aim to restore values to that child's normal levels. Do not use end-tidal CO_2 as a surrogate for $PaCO_2$ when aiming for normocapnia as part of neuroprotective care unless there is a proven correlation.

If a resuscitated child has a tracheal tube in place and starts to make a respiratory effort but remains unconscious, it is usually preferable to leave them intubated and ventilated (with appropriate sedation and analgesia) until after transfer and admission to PICU since they can deteriorate rapidly, and reintubation during transfer is extremely hazardous.

C Circulation

The aim of circulatory management is to ensure adequate organ perfusion and tissue oxygenation.

Haemodynamic function and cardiac rhythm are likely to be unstable in the immediate post-resuscitation phase. Clinical assessment of the child will help in the evaluation of any treatment response – capillary refill time, peripheral temperature, core temperature and urine output. Minimum monitoring should be in place (ECG, SpO_2, BP and end-tidal CO_2 monitoring). Serial serum lactate is used to assess the response to management strategies.

The Mean Arterial Pressure (MAP) should be targeted at or above the 50th centile for the child. An arterial line may be required to aid the titration of intravenous fluids and vasoactive drugs to achieve this.

Urine output should be appropriate for the child's age; aim for > 1 mL kg^{-1} h^{-1} in children and > 2 mL kg^{-1} h^{-1} in infants. Assessment of central venous pressure (CVP), a measure of preload (i.e. the filling volume of the heart) may also be appropriate in some children but will require insertion of a central line. After fluid resuscitation, palpation of the liver edge may also give an indication of fluid status (particularly in infants) and should normally be < 1 cm beyond the costal margin.

Assessment of the child's fluid balance and circulating volume must be considered. Resuscitation boluses of balanced crystalloids or 0.9% sodium chloride may be required to optimise circulating volume. Crystalloids can be safely used in the peri-resuscitation period, but some patients may require blood products (red cells, fresh frozen plasma, cryoprecipitate or platelets).

Maintenance fluids should be based on biochemistry evaluations, and blood glucose should be measured. Glucose should be cautiously administered as required to avoid hypoglycaemia or hyperglycaemia, as both conditions can have a deleterious effect on neurological outcome in critically unwell children. Careful monitoring is required. During the immediate post-resuscitation period, decisions about securing longer-term vascular access will be required (e.g. insertion of central venous cannulae to replace intraosseous access or additional lines to deliver specific medications).

Ongoing resuscitation of the child may necessitate vasoactive infusions, such as inotropes or vasoconstrictors. These are preferably administered via dedicated central venous catheters but can be administered peripherally in the short-term. Having a central line with multiple lumens ensures that these drugs are not interrupted to deliver other medications and fluids, and avoids incompatibilities.

Commonly used vasoactive drugs include adrenaline and noradrenaline but consensus guidelines for specific conditions should be followed (e.g. sepsis guidelines for children).

D Disability

The brain is highly vulnerable to hypoxia and ischaemia. It can be injured by direct trauma, infection, hyperglycaemia, hypoglycaemia, hypocapnia, seizures or raised intracranial pressure. Secondary brain injury can be minimised by stabilising systemic blood pressure, treating seizures, normalising blood gases (taking particular care to avoid hypoxia) and correcting glucose and electrolyte abnormalities.

Neurological status: should be performed early to obtain a post-resuscitation baseline, help identify neurological deficits and possibly help to predict prognosis.

The conscious level should be assessed with either the AVPU or Glasgow Coma Scale scoring systems. Pupil reactivity, posturing and focal signs should also be noted and regularly recorded.

Neuroprotective care post-ROSC aims to avoid secondary brain injury.

Temperature control: after ROSC, strict control of temperature to avoid hyperthermia (> 37.5°C) and severe hypothermia (< 32°C) is mandatory. Hyperthermia post cardiorespiratory arrest is common in the first 48 h and is

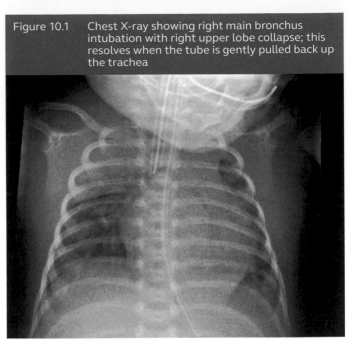

Figure 10.1   Chest X-ray showing right main bronchus intubation with right upper lobe collapse; this resolves when the tube is gently pulled back up the trachea

known to worsen brain injury with an increase in morbidity for every 1°C above 37°C; hence fever should be treated aggressively with antipyretics and active cooling.

Blood glucose: hypoglycaemia (< 3 mmol L^{-1}) and hyperglycaemia are associated with worse neurological outcome. Studies have not shown that tight control of blood glucose levels confers any benefit for paediatric patients, and it carries the risk of inadvertent hypoglycaemia, so it is not recommended. Glucose should be delivered as a continuous infusion rather than as boluses, and blood glucose levels should be monitored frequently.

E Exposure

Exposure and a full examination to detect any lesions (e.g. rashes, wounds) should be undertaken and may help in making the diagnosis, informing specific management of the child (e.g. the purpuric rash of meningococcaemia may prompt treatment with broad-spectrum antibiotics if not already given). Care should be taken to respect the child's dignity, and excessive hypothermia avoided, especially in infants.

Other organs

Renal function should be monitored by measuring urine output and the serum urea and creatinine levels. Insertion of a urinary catheter may be necessary. Treatment is directed towards maintaining an adequate circulating volume, which sustains renal perfusion. Hence diuretics are only indicated if decreased urine output persists after adequate fluid resuscitation.

The gastrointestinal mucosa and liver can also be affected by hypoxia and ischaemia. Gastrointestinal mucosal injury can contribute to multi-organ failure due to leakage of toxins and bacteria into the circulation. Treatment is aimed at maintaining adequate circulating volume and gut perfusion.

Table 10.2 Post-resuscitation investigations

Investigation	Rationale
Arterial and/or venous blood gas (plus lactate)	Ensure adequate ventilation Assess tissue perfusion
Biochemistry	Assess renal function Maintain normoglycaemia Assess electrolyte balance (especially Na^+, K^+, Mg^{2+}, Ca^+) Liver function tests to look for ischaemic injury
Full blood count Clotting screen Group and Save Cultures (blood, urine etc.)	Assess haemoglobin level and exclude anaemia Monitor infection markers (e.g. white cell count, CRP etc.) Identify underlying blood disorders Assess any coagulopathy from sepsis or ischaemia Allows for urgent crossmatch
Chest X-ray	Establish position of tracheal tube, central venous lines, gastric tube (as appropriate) Detect underlying pathology (primary respiratory or cardiac disease, aspiration) Exclude pneumothorax/rib fractures Estimate heart size
Other investigations as indicated (e.g. head CT or pelvis X-rays, cardiac echography, 12-lead ECG, serum and urine toxicology)	

Further assessment

History

A comprehensive history is important to determine the cause of cardiorespiratory arrest and plan ongoing management. This should include relevant details about the past medical history, previous health/ill health and medications, as well as precipitating events. Details about the initial management of the current event (e.g. delay in starting resuscitation) should also be sought, as these may influence ongoing management.

Investigations

The child's physiological parameters are likely to be deranged in the immediate post-resuscitation period; urgent haematological, biochemical, radiological and cardiological investigations may all be indicated (Table 10.2).

Facilitating safe patient transfer

Following cardiorespiratory stabilisation, the child should be safely transferred to an appropriate PICU for definitive and ongoing medical support. The decision to transfer should be made only after discussion between senior members of the transport/PICU team, the clinical emergency team leader and the child's primary team (if available for consultation). Other considerations pre-transfer are listed in Table 10.3.

Table 10.3 Pre-transfer considerations

Stabilise the child (ongoing or recurrent cardiorespiratory arrest precludes transfer).	
Arrange the most appropriate mode of transport.	
Inform the paediatric consultant and any other speciality lead involved in the immediate care of the child (e.g. anaesthetist, surgeon, department nurse in charge, child protection lead if appropriate).	
Inform the child's parents of transfer details and ensure they have appropriate means of transport to the PICU.	
A	Ensure a secure airway (aspirate any endotracheal tube secretions prior to transfer).
B	Ensure appropriate settings on transport ventilator, adequate portable oxygen supplies for the length of the journey, and alternative means of ventilating the child (manual ventilation circuit that can be used either with or without oxygen supply). Deflate the stomach with a gastric tube.
C	Ensure adequate intravenous access.
D	Ensure adequate sedation and analgesia being delivered +/- neuromuscular blocker and that sufficient drugs are available for the journey. Reassess pupillary reaction and conscious level.
E	Ensure heat loss during transfer is kept to a minimum (unless intentionally cooling the patient) with insulation blankets and warming devices.
Fluids: Ensure maintenance fluids are running, and blood glucose levels are monitored. Consider a urinary catheter prior to transfer. Monitor urine output. Transfer all medication/fluid infusions and monitoring to portable transport devices.	
Contact PICU to update them of the child's clinical status and provide an estimated time of arrival before departure.	
Prepare full and clear records of the event, including all interventions (copies of notes, drug charts, X-rays is ideal).	
Just prior to moving the child run through the ABCDE assessment aloud with all team members involved. Request any suggestions or comments from the team and then confirm with all team members that they are in agreement to move the patient.	

10: Summary learning

ROSC following cardiopulmonary resuscitation is merely the first step in the continuous process of resuscitation management.

The ongoing management of seriously ill children includes appropriate vital sign monitoring, supportive therapies based on continuous ABCDE assessment and safe transfer to a PICU facility.

My key take-home messages from this chapter are:

Further reading

Brierley J, Carcillo JA, Choong K et al. Clinical practice parameters for hemodynamic support of pediatric and neonatal septic shock: 2007 update from the American College of Critical Care Medicine. Critical Care Medicine 2009 37(2):666-88.

Macrae D, Grieve R, Allen E et al. A Randomised Trial of Hyperglycemic Control in Pediatric Intensive Care. New England Journal of Medicine. 2014. 370; 107-118.

Moler FW, Silverstein FS, Holubkov R et al. Therapeutic Hypothermia after Out-of-Hospital Cardiac Arrest in Children. New England Journal of Medicine. 2015. 372. 1898-1908.

Moler FW, Silverstein FS, Holubkov R et al. Therapeutic Hypothermia after In-Hospital Cardiac Arrest in Children. New England Journal of Medicine 2017;376:318-329.

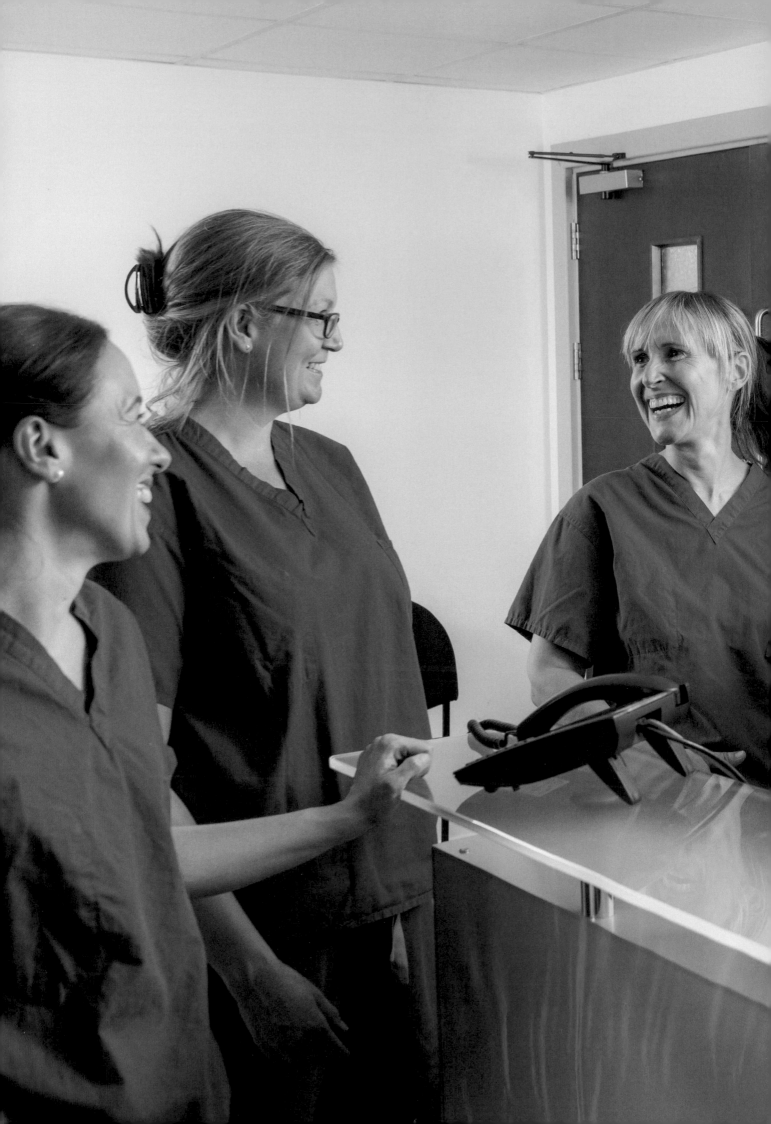

In this chapter

The learning outcomes will enable you to:

Be an effective team member and team member

Consider the role of non-technical skills during resuscitation

Effectively use structured communication tools such as SBAR and RSVP

Non-technical skills

Non-technical skills can be defined as the cognitive, social and personal resource skills that complement technical skills and contribute to safe and efficient task performance. More simply, they are the things that affect our personal performance. Non-technical skills of leadership and teamwork have been identified as important contributory factors to technical skill performance in both simulated settings and poor clinical outcomes in acute medical settings.

Paediatric resuscitation is particularly emotive, stressful and often time-critical. The skills of chest compressions, vascular access, defibrillation, and rhythm recognition are considered typically to be important aspects of paediatric resuscitation management. These are all technical skills that are learnt from books, lectures, courses and peers. Although they are important for the successful resuscitation of a child, there is another group of skills that is becoming increasingly recognised in medicine as equally important.

The importance of non-technical skills in emergencies is now widely accepted across many acute medical specialities, including surgery, anaesthesia, critical care and acute medicine. Examples of poor non-technical skills include poor communication, poor leadership, poor decision-making, and absence of clarity in role allocation, all of which can lead to system errors. Episodes of resuscitation with documented system errors are associated with poor clinical outcomes. In the context of resuscitation, which is fundamentally a team effort, the contribution of teamwork and leadership is therefore expected to make a significant contribution to patient outcome. Understanding and improving non-technical skills may help to reduce human errors, creating more effective teams and improve patient safety. An effective team leader can help focus the team members, improve team commitment and act as the role model for others.

The key non-technical skills are:

- situational awareness
- decision making
- team working
- leadership
- task management.

Situational awareness

This can be described as an individual's awareness of the environment at the moment of an event and its analysis to understand how individual actions may impact future events. This becomes particularly important when many events are happening simultaneously, for example, at a resuscitation attempt. High information input with poor situational awareness may lead to poor decision making with serious consequences. At a resuscitation, all those participating will have varying degrees of situational awareness. In a well-functioning team, all members will have a common understanding of current events or shared situational awareness. It is important that only the relevant information is shared; otherwise, there is too much distraction or noise.

Situational awareness in resuscitation will include perception of environment and events taking place, comprehension of their meaning, and future projection.

Information gathering
What are the potential causes of cardiac arrest?
- location of arrest
- information from staff about events leading up to the arrest
- note the actions already initiated
- confirm who is present, names, skills, roles and who is leading.

Interpretation
What immediate steps are needed?
- confirm diagnosis
- checking that a monitor has been attached and interpreting what it shows
- determine immediate needs and necessary actions.

Future planning
What are the next steps?
- consider the impact of interventions
- plan for next steps.

Decision making

This is defined as the cognitive process of choosing a specific course of action from several alternatives. At a resuscitation, the many decisions to be made usually fall to the team leader. The leader will assimilate information from the team members and from personal observation and will use this to determine appropriate interventions and shares these with the team. Typical decisions made at a resuscitation may include:

- likely reversible causes of the arrest
- appropriate treatment such as drugs or airway management
- how long to continue resuscitation
- appropriate post-resuscitation care.

Once a decision has been made, clear unambiguous communication with the team members is essential to ensure that it is implemented.

Team working

This is one of the most important non-technical skills that contribute to the successful management of critical situations. A team is a group of individuals working together with a common goal or purpose. In a team, the members usually have complementary skills and, through coordination of effort, work synergistically. Teams work best when everyone knows each other's name, when they are doing something they perceive to be important, and when their role is within their experience and competence. Optimal team function mandates a team leader.

There are several characteristics of a good resuscitation team member:

- **Competence** – has the skills required at a resuscitation and performs them to the best of their ability.
- **Commitment** – strives to achieve the best outcome for the patient.
- **Communicates openly** – is able to articulate their findings and actions taken, raises concerns about clinical or safety issues, and listens to briefings and instructions.
- **Supportive** – enables others to achieve their best.
- **Accountable** – for their own and the team's actions.
- **Prepared to admit when help is needed.**
- **Creative** – suggests different ways of interpreting the situation.
- **Participates in providing feedback.**

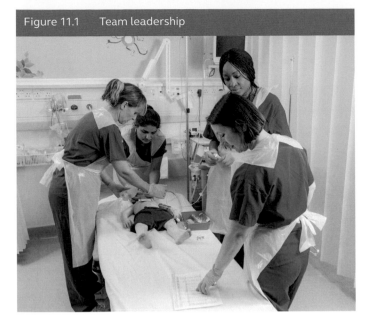

Figure 11.1   Team leadership

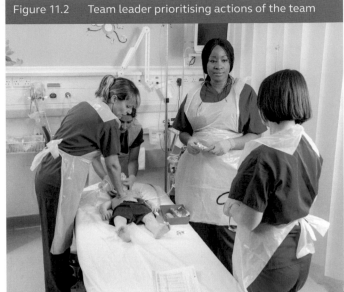

Figure 11.2   Team leader prioritising actions of the team

Team leadership

A team leader provides guidance, direction and instruction to the team members to enable successful completion of their stated objective (Figure 11.1). They lead by example and integrity. Team leaders need experience, not simply seniority. Team leadership can be considered a process; with training, it is available to everyone within the team and not restricted to those with leadership traits.

There are several attributes recognisable in a good team leader:

- knows everyone in the team by name and knows their capability
- accepts the leadership role
- is able to delegate tasks appropriately (preferably before the event)
- is knowledgeable and has sufficient credibility to influence the team through role modelling and professionalism
- recognises their own limitations and asks for support from the team
- is a good communicator – not just good at giving instructions, but is a good listener and decisive in action
- stays calm, keeps everyone focused and controls distractions
- is empathetic towards the whole team
- is assertive and authoritative when required
- shows tolerance towards hesitancy or nervousness in the emergency setting
- has good situational awareness; able to constantly monitor the situation, with an up-to-date overview, listening and deciding on a course of action.

During a cardiorespiratory arrest, the role of the team leader is not always immediately obvious. The leader should clarify early on that they are assuming the role of team leader.

Specifically, at a cardiorespiratory arrest, the leader should:

- follow current resuscitation guidelines or explain a reason for any significant deviation from standard protocols
- consult with the team or call for senior advice and assistance if unsure about an intervention
- play to the strengths of team members and allow them some autonomy if their skills are adequate
- allocate roles and tasks throughout the resuscitation and be specific; this avoids several people or nobody attempting the task!
- uses the two minute cycles of chest compressions to plan tasks and safety aspects of the resuscitation attempt with the team
- thanks the team at the end of the resuscitation attempt and ensures that staff and relatives are being supported
- completes all documentation and ensures an adequate handover.

Task management

During the resuscitation of a child, either in full cardiorespiratory arrest or peri-arrest, there are numerous tasks to be carried out by the team members, either sequentially or simultaneously. Cognitive aids such as a checklist or easy access guidelines could be used as support but will need a dedicated team member to read and check them. The coordination and control, or management, of these tasks is the responsibility of the team leader (Figure 11.2).

Tasks can include:

- identifying the resources required - ensuring that equipment is checked and specifics organised and delegated
- being inclusive of all team members

- being prepared for both the expected and the unexpected
- prioritising actions of the team
- watching out for fatigue, stress and distress amongst the team.
- managing conflict
- communicating with relatives
- communicating with experts for safe handover both by telephone and in person
- debriefing the team
- reporting untoward incidents, particularly equipment or system failures
- participating in audit.

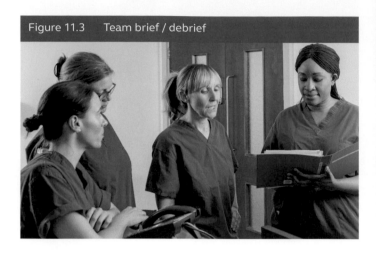

Figure 11.3   Team brief / debrief

The importance of communication when managing a sick child

Communication problems are a factor in up to 80% of adverse incidents or near-miss reports in hospitals. This failure of communication is also evident when a medical emergency occurs on a ward and a doctor or nurse summons senior help. The call for help is often suboptimal, with failure by the caller to communicate the seriousness of the situation and convey information to inform the recipient of the urgency of the situation. The poor-quality information heightens the anxiety of the person responding to the call, who is then uncertain of the nature of the problem they are about to face.

A well-structured process that is simple, reliable, and dependable will enable the caller to convey important facts and urgency and help the recipient plan ahead. It was for similar reasons that the ABCDE approach was developed as an aide-memoire of the key technical skills required to manage seriously ill/deteriorating patients.

The use of the SBAR (Situation, Background, Assessment, Recommendation) or RSVP (Reason, Story, Vital signs, Plan) tool enables effective, timely communication between individuals from different clinical backgrounds and hierarchies (Table 11.1).

Resuscitation teams

The resuscitation team may take the form of a traditional cardiorespiratory arrest team which is called only when a cardiorespiratory arrest is recognised. Alternatively, hospitals may have strategies to recognise patients at risk of deterioration and to summon a team (e.g. medical emergency team) before cardiorespiratory arrest occurs.

The term 'resuscitation team' reflects a range of immediate response teams. The resuscitation team may change daily or more frequently, and members may not know each other or the skill mix within the team. The team should, therefore meet ('huddle') at the beginning of their period on duty to introduce themselves and allocate roles (Figure 11.3).

Preparation

During the 'huddle', the team will identify a team leader who will pre-allocate core tasks according to the number of team members available and the skill mix, these include:

- airway management and ventilation
- pulse check and chest compressions
- attaching monitoring and/or defibrillation
- obtaining IO/IV access, preparing and administering drugs
- recording events.

Relatives can be looked after by another member of the team; this should not be the most junior member of staff as parents need a careful explanation of the events.

Clinical staff who participate as members of the resuscitation team must be up to date with advanced skills in paediatric life support and must be familiar with the local equipment.

It is also important that resuscitation teams practice skills together to try to avoid errors. This may involve high and low-fidelity scenarios on courses such as EPALS and involve on-site 'mock' clinical emergencies.

Team debrief

Every effort should be made to enable the team members to meet to debrief (e.g. difficulties or concerns about their performance, problems or concerns with equipment), and submit incident reports). Debriefing has been shown to enhance team performance. It may also be possible to carry out a formal handover to the incoming team.

Table 11.1 SBAR (Situation, Background, Assessment, Recommendation) **and RSVP** (Reason, Story, Vital signs, Plan)

SBAR	RSVP	Content	Example
Situation	**Reason**	Introduce yourself and check you are speaking to the correct person. Identify the patient you are calling about (who and where). Say what you think the current problem is, or appears to be. State what you need advice about. Useful phrases: • The problem appears to be cardiac/respiratory/neurological/sepsis. • I'm not sure what the problem is but the patient is deteriorating. • The patient is unstable, getting worse and I need help.	*Hi, I'm Dr Smith the paediatric F2.* *I am calling about Sam Brown on the paediatric ward who I think has a severe pneumonia and is septic.* *They have an oxygen saturation of 90% despite high-flow oxygen and I am very worried.*
Background	**Story**	Background information about the patient. Reason for admission. Relevant past medical history.	*They are 6 years old and previously fit and well.* *They have had a fever and a cough for 2 days.* *They were admitted yesterday.*
Assessment	**Vital signs**	Include specific observations and vital sign values based on ABCDE approach. • Airway • Breathing • Circulation • Disability • Exposure • The PEWS score is…	*They look very unwell and are tiring* *Airway – they can say a few words* *Breathing – their respiratory rate is 34, with widespread wheeze in both lung fields and has bronchial breathing on the left side. Their oxygen saturation is 90% on high-flow oxygen. I am getting a blood gas and chest X-ray* *Circulation – their pulse is 180, and blood pressure is 90/60* *Disability – they are drowsy and clinging onto their mum* *Exposure – there are no rashes*
Recommendation	**Plan**	State explicitly what you want the person you are calling to do. What by when? Useful phrases: • I am going to start the following treatment; is there anything else you can suggest? • I am going to do the following investigations; is there anything else you can suggest? • If they do not improve; when would you like to be called? • I don't think I can do anymore; I would like you to see the patient urgently.	*They are only on oral antibiotics so I am starting an IV* *I need help – please can you come straight away?*

Quality and audit

The Institute of Medicine defines that quality care is safe, effective, patient-centred, timely, efficient and equitable. Hospitals, resuscitation teams and EPALS providers should ensure they deliver these aspects of quality to improve the care of the deteriorating child and children in cardiorespiratory arrest. Two aspects of this are safety incident reporting (also called adverse or critical incident reporting) and collecting good quality data.

Audit and outcome after cardiorespiratory arrest

Most modern defibrillators allow the cardiorespiratory arrest management to be downloaded with a timeline of different rhythms and actions taken in terms of defibrillation, cardioversion and cardiopulmonary resuscitation. It also allows the quality of CPR delivered to be reviewed when a feedback device has been used.

Locally, this useful information can help teams use reflection and feedback to improve future performance, especially in terms of adherence to resuscitation guidelines, the percentage of time CPR has been performed and 'hands-off' time.

National audit of resuscitation processes and outcomes provides information about whether interventions and changes made to resuscitation guidelines improve patient care. New interventions that improve survival rate even marginally are important because of the many individuals who suffer a cardiorespiratory arrest each year. Local hospitals or healthcare systems are unlikely to have sufficient patients to identify these effects or eliminate confounders.

Therefore, resuscitation outcome and processes should be reported in a standard manner to allow comparison between different areas of practice. The internationally agreed Utstein template is a standardised system of reporting that allows the comparison of resuscitation data across different countries and healthcare systems. This facilitates the use of large national and multi-national databases to evaluate the impact of new drugs or techniques.

National Cardiac Arrest Audit (NCAA)

In the UK, the National Cardiac Arrest Audit (NCAA) is an ongoing, national, comparative outcome audit of in-hospital cardiorespiratory arrests (Table 11.2). It is a joint initiative between Resuscitation Council UK and the Intensive Care National Audit & Research Centre (ICNARC) and is open to all acute hospitals in the UK and Ireland. The audit monitors and reports on the incidence of, and outcome from, in-hospital cardiorespiratory arrest (following a 2222 call) to inform practice and policy. It aims to identify and foster improvements in the prevention, care delivery and outcomes from cardiorespiratory arrest. Data are collected according to standardised definitions and entered onto the NCAA secure web-based system. Once data are validated, hospitals are provided with activity reports and comparative reports, allowing a comparison to be made within hospitals and between hospitals locally, nationally, and internationally. Furthermore, NCAA enables the monitoring of the effects of new guidelines, drugs, techniques etc., that would not be possible on a hospital-by-hospital basis.

Table 11.2   Outcomes following in-hospital cardiac arrest (UK) for children in participating hospitals January 2012 to December 2018 NCAA data. Total number Cardiac arrests = 1580

	VF/pVT	Asystole	PEA	Bradycardia
% of arrests*	4.3%	22.2 %	30.3%	29.7%
% ROSC > 20 mins	75%	55.9%	55.9%	87%
% hospital discharge	63.9%	41%	41%	70.6%
Overall survival to hospital discharge (all events)	54.2 %	54.2 %	54.2 %	54.2 %

11: Summary learning

Non-technical skills are important during resuscitation.

Use SBAR or RSVP for effective communication.

My key take-home messages from this chapter are:

Further reading

Andersen PO, Jensen MK, Lippert A, et al.: Identifying non-technical skills and barriers for improvement of teamwork in cardiac arrest teams. Resuscitation 2010; 81:695–702.

Cooper S, Cant R, Porter J, et al.: Rating medical emergency teamwork performance: Development of the Team Emergency Assessment Measure (TEAM). Resuscitation 2010; 81:446–452.

Featherstone P, Chalmers T, Smith GB. RSVP: a system for communication of deterioration in hospital patients. Br J Nurs 2008;17:860-64.

Flin R, O'Connor P, Crichton M. Safety at the Sharp End: a Guide to Non- Technical Skills. Aldershot: Ashgate, 2008.

Peltonen V, Peltonen LM, Salantera S et al. An observational study of technical and non-technical skills in advanced life support in the clinical setting. Resuscitation 2020; 53:162-168

Yeung J, Ong G, Davies R, Gao F, Perkins GDP. Factors affecting team leadership skills and their relationship with quality of cardiopulmonary resuscitation. Crit Care Med 2012; 40:2617–2621.

Skellett S, Orzechowska I, Thomas K, Fortune PM. The Landscape of paediatric in-hospital cardiac arrest in the United Kingdom National Cardiac Arrest Audit. Resuscitation. 2020 Oct;155:165-171

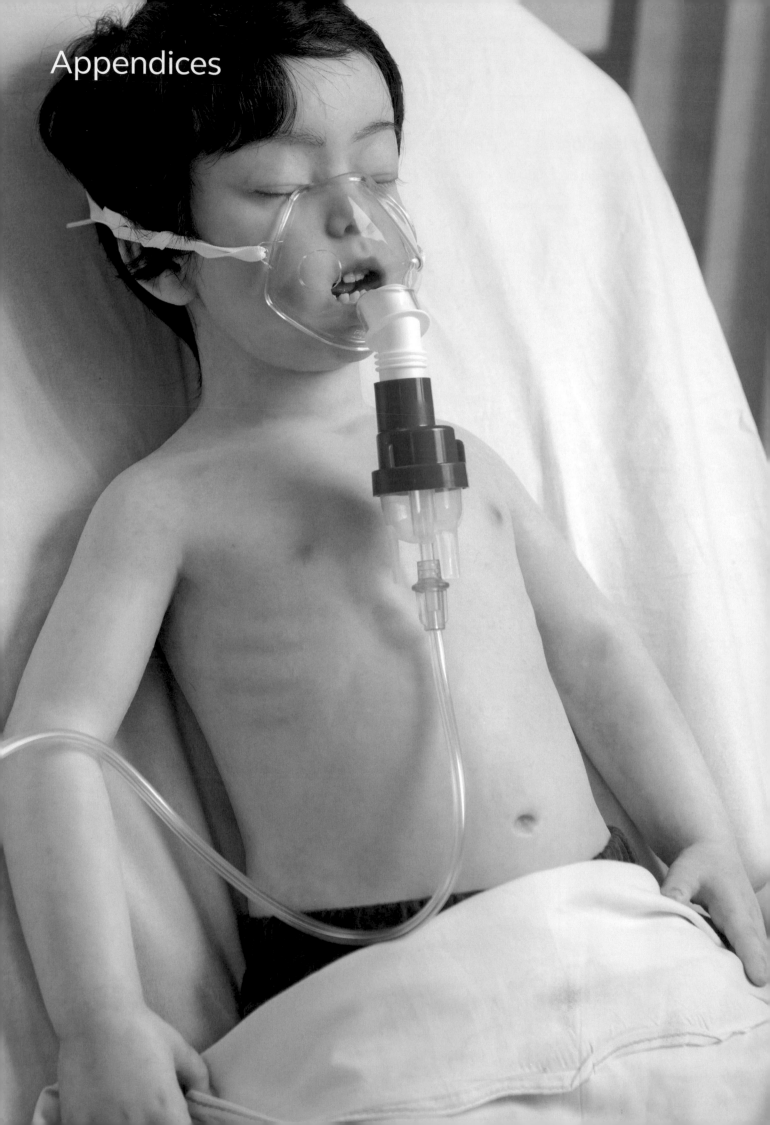

Appendices

Appendix A
Paediatric emergency drug chart

Age	Weight kg	Adrenaline 1:10 000 — 10 mcg kg⁻¹ — IV, IO (mL)	Fluid bolus — Balanced isotonic crystalloid OR 0.9% Saline — 10 mL kg⁻¹ — IV, IO (mL)	Glucose 10% — 2 mL kg⁻¹ — IV, IO (mL) (recheck glucose after dose and repeat as required)	Sodium bicarbonate 4.2% — 1 mmol kg⁻¹ — IV, IO, UVC (mL)	Sodium bicarbonate 8.4% — 1 mmol kg⁻¹ — IV, IO (mL)	Tracheal tube Uncuffed (ID mm)	Tracheal tube Cuffed — Monitor cuff pressure (ID mm)	Defibrillation 4 joules kg⁻¹ Monophasic or biphasic Manual
< 1 month	3.5	0.35	35	7	7	–	3.0	–	20
1 month	4	0.4	40	8	8	–	3.0–3.5	3.0	20
3 months	5	0.5	50	10	10	–	3.5	3.0	20
6 months	7	0.7	70	14	–	–	3.5	3.0	30
1 year	10	1.0	100	20	–	10	4.0	3.5	40
2 years	12	1.2	120	24	–	12	4.5	4.0	50
3 years	14	1.4	140	28	–	14	4.5–5.0	4.0–4.5	60
4 years	16	1.6	160	32	–	16	5.0	4.5	60
5 years	18	1.8	180	36	–	18	5.0–5.5	4.5–5.0	70
6 years	20	2.0	200	40	–	20	5.5	5.0	80
7 years	23	2.3	230	46	–	23	5.5–6.0	5.0–5.5	100
8 years	26	2.6	260	50	–	26	–	6.0–6.5	100
10 years	30	3.0	300	50	–	30	–	7.0	120
12 years	38	3.8	380	50	–	38	–	7–7.5	120
14 years	50	5.0	500	50	–	50	–	7–8	120–150
Adolescent	50	5.0	500	50	–	50	–	7–8	120–150
Adult	70	10.0	500	50	–	50	–	7–8	120–150

Notes (Fluid bolus): Consider warmed fluids
Notes (Glucose): For known hypoglycaemia

Drug	Notes
Cardioversion	Synchronised Shock, 1.0 joules kg⁻¹ escalating to 2.0 joules kg⁻¹ if unsuccessful.
Amiodarone	5 mg kg⁻¹ IV or IO bolus in arrest after 3rd and 5th shocks. Flush line with 0.9% saline or 5% glucose (max dose 300 mg).
Atropine	20 mcg kg⁻¹, maximum dose 600 mcg.
Calcium gluconate 10%	0.5 mL kg⁻¹ for hypocalcaemia, hyperkalaemia (max dose 20 mL); IV over 2–5 min if unstable, over 15–20 min if stable.
Lorazepam	100 mcg kg⁻¹ IV or IO for treatment of seizures. Can be repeated after 10 min. Maximum single dose 4 mg.
Adenosine	IV or IO for treatment of SVT: 150 mcg kg⁻¹ (0–11 months of age); 100 mcg kg⁻¹ (1–11 years of age) Increase dose in steps 50–100 mcg kg⁻¹ every 1–2 min for repeat doses. 12–17 years: 3 mg, followed by 6 mg after 1–2 min if required, followed by 12 mg after 1–2 min if required. Requires large saline flush and ECG monitoring.
Anaphylaxis	Adrenaline 1:1000 IM: < 6 months 100–150 mcg (0.1–0.15 mL), 6 months–6 years 150 mcg (0.15 mL), 6–12 years 300 mcg (0.3 mL), > 12 years 500 mcg (0.5 mL); can be repeated after 5 min. After 2 IM injections treat as refractory anaphylaxis and start low dose adrenaline infusion IV.

- Weights averaged on lean body mass from 50th centile weights for males and females.
- Drug doses based on Resuscitation Council UK Guidelines 2021 recommendations.
- Recommendations for tracheal tubes are based on full term neonates.
- For newborns glucose at 2.5 mL kg⁻¹ is recommended.

Anaphylaxis

Anaphylaxis?

| A = Airway | B = Breathing | C = Circulation | D = Disability | E = Exposure |

Diagnosis – look for:

- Sudden onset of Airway and/or Breathing and/or Circulation problems[1]
- And usually skin changes (e.g. itchy rash)

Call for HELP
Call resuscitation team or ambulance

- Remove trigger if possible (e.g. stop any infusion)
- Lie patient flat (with or without legs elevated)
  - A sitting position may make breathing easier
  - If pregnant, lie on left side

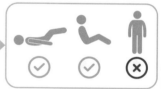

Give intramuscular (IM) adrenaline[2]

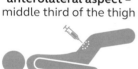

Inject at **anterolateral aspect** – middle third of the thigh

- Establish airway
- Give high flow oxygen
- Apply monitoring: pulse oximetry, ECG, blood pressure

If no response:

- Repeat IM adrenaline after 5 minutes
- IV fluid bolus[3]

If no improvement in Breathing or Circulation problems[1] despite TWO doses of IM adrenaline:

- Confirm resuscitation team or ambulance has been called
- Follow REFRACTORY ANAPHYLAXIS ALGORITHM

---

1. Life-threatening problems

Airway
Hoarse voice, stridor

Breathing
↑work of breathing, wheeze, fatigue, cyanosis, $SpO_2 < 94\%$

Circulation
Low blood pressure, signs of shock, confusion, reduced consciousness

2. Intramuscular (IM) adrenaline
Use adrenaline at 1 mg/mL (1:1000) concentration

Adult and child > 12 years:	500 micrograms IM (0.5 mL)
Child 6–12 years:	300 micrograms IM (0.3 mL)
Child 6 months to 6 years:	150 micrograms IM (0.15 mL)
Child < 6 months:	100–150 micrograms IM (0.1–0.15 mL)

The above doses are for IM injection **only**.
Intravenous adrenaline for anaphylaxis to be given **only by experienced specialists** in an appropriate setting.

3. IV fluid challenge
Use crystalloid

Adults:	500–1000 mL
Children:	10 mL/kg

Acute asthma in children

Acute asthma in children aged 2–12 years

These clinical features increase the probability of a diagnosis of asthma:

- More than one of the following: wheeze, cough, difficulty breathing and chest tightness. The risk is increased if these symptoms are recurrent, worse at night or in the early morning, occur during or after exercise or trigger dependent (e.g. with exposure to pets, cold, humidity, heightened emotions or occurring independent of upper respiratory tract infections).
- Personal history of atopic disorder.
- Family history of atopic disorder and/or asthma.
- Widespread wheeze heard on auscultation.
- History of improvement in symptoms or lung function in response to adequate therapy.

Acute asthma in children under 2 years

The assessment of acute asthma in early childhood can be difficult.

- Intermittent wheezing attacks are usually due to viral infection and the response to asthma medication is inconsistent.
- Prematurity and low birth weight are risk factors for recurrent wheezing.
- The differential diagnosis of symptoms includes: aspiration pneumonitis, pneumonia, bronchiolitis, tracheomalacia, complications of underlying conditions such as congenital anomalies and cystic fibrosis.

Classification of severity of acute presentation

Moderate asthma

Normal mental state

Ability to talk in sentences or vocalise as normal

Some accessory muscle use

PEF ≥ 50% of best or predicted

O_2 saturations > 92% in air

Moderate tachycardia

HR ≤ 125 min^{-1} (> 5 years)

HR ≤ 140 min^{-1} (2–5 years)

RR ≤ 30 min^{-1} (> 5 years)

RR ≤ 40 min^{-1} (2–5 years)

Management

Continuous O_2 saturation monitoring

High-flow O_2 via face mask titrated to achieve O_2 saturations 94–98%

ß2 agonist 2–10 puffs via pMDI + spacer

+/-face mask, repeat dose every 20 min reviewing effect; no improvement in 1 h treat as acute severe

Ipratropium bromide given early via pMDI

+ spacer +/- face mask, particularly if poorly responsive to ß2 agonist

Oral steroids: prednisolone 20 mg for children aged 2 to 5 years; 30 to 40 mg for children > 5 years

Acute severe asthma

Agitated, distressed

Can't complete sentences in one breath

Moderate to marked accessory muscle use

PEF 33–50% of best or predicted

O_2 saturations < 92% in air

HR > 125 min^{-1} (> 5 years)

HR > 140 min^{-1} (2–5 years)

RR > 30 min^{-1} (> 5 years)

RR > 40 min^{-1} (2–5 years)

Management

Continuous O_2 saturation monitoring

High-flow O_2 via face mask titrated to achieve O_2 saturations 94–98%

ß2 agonist nebulised (salbutamol 2.5–5 mg) every 20 min with Ipratropium bromide (250 mcg) for first 2 h; review frequently

Oral steroids: 20 mg prednisolone for children aged 2 to 5 years; 30 to 40 mg for children > 5 years

Consider intravenous magnesium and aminophylline if if the child is unresponsive to maximal doses of bronchodilators and steroids

Consider ABG if poor response to early treatment

Refer to PICU

Life-threatening asthma

Confused, drowsy, exhausted

Unable to talk

Maximal accessory muscle use (poor respiratory effort is **pre-terminal**)

Marked tachycardia (sudden fall in HR is **pre-terminal**)

PEF < 33% of best or predicted

O_2 saturations < 92% in air

Silent chest

Cyanosis

Hypotension

Management

Continuous O_2 saturation monitoring

High-flow O_2 via face mask titrated to achieve O_2 saturations 94–98%

Refer to PICU

ß2 agonist nebulised (salbutamol 2.5–5 mg) every 20 min with Ipratropium bromide (250 mcg) for first 2 h; review frequently

Oral steroids: 20 mg prednisolone (2–5 years); 30 to 40 mg (> 5 years). Repeat dose if vomiting or consider intravenous steroids (hydrocortisone 4 mg kg^{-1} every 4 h)

Give bolus of intravenous magnesium.

Consider early single bolus dose of IV salbutamol where child has responded poorly to inhaled therapy followed by an infusion

Consider aminophylline if child unresponsive to maximal doses of bronchodilators and steroids

Consider ABG if poor response to early treatment.

pMDI – pressurised metered-dose inhalers

Note: Evidence is unclear which of intravenous salbutamol, aminophylline or magnesium should be the first line in severe asthma.

Early management of asthma – September 2019. Based on the British Thoracic Society, Scottish Intercollegiate Guidelines Network, British guideline on the management of asthma revised 2019

Appendix D
Treating convulsive status epilepticus in children

SEIZURE STARTS

Management

- Confirm clinically
- Check ABC, high-flow O_2, attach monitoring
- Check blood glucose, treat < 3 mmol L^{-1}

5 MIN

1st line agents

- Consider pre-hospital treatment already given: 2 doses of benzodiazepines max
- **Midazolam** 0.3–0.5 mg kg^{-1} bucally – see BNFc for exact age related dose
OR
- **Lorazepam** 0.1 mg kg^{-1} IV or IO

10–15 MIN

- **Lorazepam** 0.1 mg kg^{-1} IV
- Reconfirm epileptic seizure and prepare second-line agent of choice for next step

15–35 MIN

2nd line agents

- **Levetiracetam** 30–60 mg kg^{-1} (over 5 min, max 3 g)
OR
- **Phenytoin** 20 mg kg^{-1} by slow IV infusion over 20 min with ECG monitoring
OR
- **Phenobarbital** 20 mg kg^{-1} by IV infusion over 5 min

Call anaesthetist and PICU

20–40 MIN

2nd or 3rd line agents

- If preparation for deeper anaethesia with I+V complete, proceed to next step
OR
- Administer further alternative second-line drug (levetiracetam, phenytoin, phenobarbitol)

3rd line agents

- Rapid sequence induction of anaesthesia using thiopental sodium 4 mg kg^{-1} IV
OR
- Propofol 1–1.5 mg kg^{-1} IV (with single dose recuronium if using NMB); ketamine and midazolam alternatives
- Intubation and ventilation; monitoring neurological signs
- Ongoing seizures are not always easy to identify (EEG)

- Definition of convulsive status epilepticus (CSE) is a seizure that continues for greater than 5 min, so treatment usually starts once seizure has lasted > 5 min
- After 5 min seizures are unlikely to spontaneously terminate
- The risk of a seizure becoming refractory increases with increasing seizure duration.
- *ESETT/**ECLIPSE/***ConSEPT trials showed equal potency for phenytoin, levetiracetam and valproate
- Levetiracetam has a good safety profile and is easy to administer
- Children who frequently have seizures or CSE usually have an individually tailored guideline.
- Do not give phenytoin too rapidly as it will cause bradycardia and/or asystole.
- In sepsis consider measuring calcium and magnesium levels as they are sometimes low.
- Monitor glucose aim for 4-8 mmol L^{-1}
- Measure serum sodium and treat if < 125 mmol L^{-1} (3 mL kg^{-1} 3% sodium chloride)
- Consider temperature control measures if hyperthermic
- Consider meningitis, encephalitis and Raised ICP
- Consider CNS haemorrhage if signs of trauma
- There is no evidence for the ideal third line agent: thiopentone, propofol, ketamine and midazolam may all be used

* Kapur et al. Randomized Trial of Three Anticonvulsant Medications for Status Epilepticus. N Engl J Med 2019;381:2103-2113.doi:10.1056/NEJMoa1905795

** Lyttle M, Pereira M et al. Levetiracetam versus phenytoin for second-line treatment of paediatric convulsive status epilepticus (EcLiPSE): a multicentre, open-label, randomised trial. Lancet, Volume 393, Issue 10186, 2125 – 2134

*** Dalziel SR, Borland ML et al; PREDICT research network. Levetiracetam versus phenytoin for second-line treatment of convulsive status epilepticus in children (Concept): an open-label, multicentre, randomised controlled trial. Lancet. 2019 May 25;393(10186):2135-2145

Emergency Paediatric Tracheostomy Management

SAFETY - STIMULATE - SHOUT FOR HELP - OXYGEN

SAFE:	**Check Safe area, Stimulate, and Shout for help**
AIRWAY:	**Open child's airway:** head tilt / chin lift / pillow or towel under shoulders may help
OXYGEN:	Ensure **high flow oxygen** to the **tracheostomy AND the face** as soon as oxygen available
CAPNOGRAPHY:	Exhaled carbon dioxide waveform may indicate a patent airway (advanced response)

Basic Response

SUCTION TO ASSESS TRACHEOSTOMY PATENCY

Remove attachments: humidifier (HME), speaking valve
Change inner tube (if present)
Inner tubes may need re-inserting to connect to breathing circuits

Can you pass a SUCTION catheter?

The tracheostomy tube is patent
Perform tracheal suction
Consider partial obstruction

Yes → **CONTINUE ASSESSMENT (ABCDE)**

No →

EMERGENCY TRACHEOSTOMY TUBE CHANGE

Deflate cuff (if present). Reassess patency after any tube change
1st change – same size tube
2nd change – one-half size smaller tube
3rd change - over suction catheter to guide

IF UNSUCCESSFUL – REMOVE THE TUBE

IS THE PATIENT BREATHING? - Look, listen and feel at the mouth and tracheostomy/stoma

No →

CALL FOR HELP: 2222 in hospital, 999 in community

5 RESCUE BREATHS

Patent Upper Airway – use the nose/mouth
Obstructed Upper Airway – use the tracheostomy/stoma

NO SIGNS OF LIFE? START CPR

15 compressions : 2 rescue breaths
Ensure help or resuscitation team called

Yes →

Continue oxygen
Stabilize
Reassess
Review

Plan for definitive airway if tube change failure

Advanced Response

Primary emergency oxygenation

Standard **ORAL airway** manoeuvres
Cover the stoma (swabs / hand).
Use:
  Bag-valve-face mask
  Oral or nasal airway adjuncts
  Supraglottic Airway (SGA)
  e.g. Laryngeal Mask Airway (LMA)

Tracheostomy STOMA ventilation
  Paediatric face-mask applied to stoma
  SGA applied to stoma

Secondary emergency oxygenation

ORAL intubation with endotracheal tube
Uncut tube, advanced beyond stoma
One half-size smaller than tracheostomy tube
'Difficult Airway' Expert and Equipment*

Attempt **intubation of STOMA**
3.0 ID tracheostomy or endotracheal tube
'Difficult Airway' Expert and Equipment*

***EQUIPMENT: Fibreoptic scope, bougie, airway exchange catheter, Airway trolley**

NTSP (Paediatric Working Group) www.tracheostomy.org.uk Review January 2022

Appendix F
Paediatric cardiac arrythmia

Assess with ABCDE approach – recognise and treat reversible causes
Oxygen if SpO$_2$ < 94%, respiratory rate, heart rate, CRT, cardiac monitoring, blood pressure, vascular access, AVPU

Signs of circulation?

NO → Follow ADVANCED LIFE SUPPORT ALGORITHM

YES

Compensated
Normal LOC, +/- respiratory distress and signs of circulatory compromise, BP > 5th centile*

Monitor for clinical deterioration and seek expert help

Treat the cause:
If bradycardia, consider oxygenation and vagal tone
If SVT, consider vagal manoeuvres
Reassess
Consider adenosine

Decompensated – seek expert help
Signs of vital organ perfusion compromise:
Reduced LOC, tachypnoea, bradycardia /tachycardia, BP < 5th centile*, CRT > 2 secs, weak or impalpable peripheral pulses

Bradycardia
< 1 year < 80 min^{-1}
> 1 year < 60 min^{-1}

Optimal oxygenation with positive pressure ventilation if required

If unconscious and HR < 60 min^{-1} despite oxygenation, start chest compressions

No response to oxygenation:
If vagal stimulation possible cause – atropine
If no response to oxygenation or atropine consider adrenaline

Pacing – very rarely required and guided by aetiology.

Tachycardia

Narrow complex

Sinus tachycardia
Infant typically 180–220 min^{-1}
Child typically 160–180 min^{-1}
Gradual onset

Treat the cause:
Physiological response:
- Crying
- Exercise
- Anxiety/fear
- Pain

Identify precipitant
Compensatory mechanism:
- Respiratory/circulatory failure
- Hypovolaemia
- Sepsis
- Anaemia

SVT
Infant > 220 min^{-1}
Child > 180 min^{-1}
Abrupt onset

Synchronised cardioversion with appropriate sedation + analgesia (e.g. IM/intranasal ketamine if delay in IV access)
Chemical cardioversion may be 1st choice if suitable IV access is in place and delay in synchronised cardioversion.
Adenosine
Consider amiodarone before 3rd shock

Broad complex

VT
Could be VT or SVT, if unsure treat as VT

If conscious:
Synchronised cardioversion with appropriate sedation + analgesia (e.g. IM/intranasal ketamine if delay in IV access, *do not delay cardioversion*).

If unconscious:
Immediate synchronised cardioversion
Consider amiodarone before 3rd shock

Drug	Atropine	Adrenaline	Adenosine	Amiodarone	Synchronised cardioversion	Magnesium
Treatment	**Up to 11 years:** 20 mcg kg^{-1}. **12–17 years:** 300–600 mcg, larger doses may be used in emergency.	**For bradycardia:** 10 mcg kg^{-1} repeat if necessary.	**Up to 1 year:** 150 mcg kg^{-1}, increase 50–100 mcg kg^{-1} every 1–2 min. Maximum single dose: Neonates 300 mcg kg^{-1}, Infants 500 mcg kg^{-1}). **1–11 years:** 100 mcg kg^{-1} increase 50–100 mcg kg^{-1} every 1–2 min. Maximum single dose: 500 mcg kg^{-1} (max. 12 mg). **12–17 years:** 3 mg IV, if required increase to 6 mg after 1–2 min, then 12 mg after 1–2 min	5 mg kg^{-1} – by SLOW IV infusion (> 20 min) before 3rd cardioversion in discussion with paediatric cardiologist/expert	With appropriate sedation + analgesia (e.g. IM/intranasal Ketamine if delay in IV access + airway management) – IV access attempts must not delay cardioversion. **1st shock:** 1 J kg^{-1}. **2nd shock:** 2 J kg^{-1}, consider up to 4 J kg^{-1}	25–50 mg kg^{-1} Maximum per dose 2 g to be given over 10–15 min, may be repeated once if necessary, in Torsades de pointes VT

Age	*Systolic BP 5th centile mmHg
1 month	50
1 year	70
5 years	75
10 years	80

RECOGNITION

Assess with ABCDE approach

A, B assessment
- Airway, RR, work of breathing, oxygen saturations, breath sounds, recognition respiratory distress/failure.
- Open airway and start high-flow O_2 15 L min^{-1} or BMV as appropriate.

C assessment
- HR, CRT, BP, peripheral and central perfusion, rhythm recognition; recognition circulatory failure/shock.
- Establish IV/IO access (take blood cultures, full blood count, blood glucose, urea and electrolytes, lactate*, blood gas and other bloods as indicated**) and give fluid resuscitation as below.

D assessment
- AVPU score; recognition of altered mental status secondary to poor perfusion.

E assessment
- Rash, temperature (high or low).

Sepsis is diagnosed if there is evidence of infection as cause of the acute illness (suspected or proven) plus at least two of the following: core temperature < 36°C or > 38.5°C; white cell count elevated or depressed for age; inappropriate tachycardia; altered mental state; reduced peripheral perfusion.

10–15 MIN

Initial resuscitation

- If no signs fluid overload (hepatomegaly, crackles at lung bases) then give 10 mL kg^{-1} balanced crystalloids*** IV bolus over 5–10 min and re-assess after each bolus up to 40–60 mL kg^{-1} or until perfusion improved.
- Therapeutic end points: CRT < 2 s; normal BP for age; UO > 1 mL kg^{-1} h^{-1}, normal pulses, normal mental state.
- Watch for signs of fluid overload; if present stop bolus therapy and start inotropic support.
- Correct hypoglycaemia and hypocalcaemia.
- Start broad-spectrum antibiotics; seek and aggressively control any infection source.
- Call for more senior help and an anaesthetist urgently; call PICU for bed +/- PICU transfer team.
- If mechanical ventilation is required, then cardiovascular instability during intubation is less likely after appropriate cardiovascular resuscitation.

15–60 MIN

Fluid refractory shock?

Start IV/IO inotrope infusion; central (preferable) or peripheral IV (clinical signs unreliable at differentiating 'warm' and 'cold' shock in children).

Adrenaline 0.05–0.3 mcg kg^{-1} min^{-1} (use more dilute infusion if peripheral)

and/or

Noradrenaline via central IV or IO, starting infusion rate 0.05 mcg kg^{-1} min^{-1}

Titrate inotropes upwards according to clinical response and haemodynamic effects using haemodynamic monitoring (where possible)****

Use ketamine +/- atropine IV/IO/IM to gain central access and airway if needed.

Fluid and catecholamine-resistant shock?

Further management as per Paediatric Intensive Care/retrieval service advice.

Warm shock – high cardiac output with low systemic vascular resistance.	**Cold shock** – low cardiac output with high systemic vascular resistance.	**Fluid in mL kg^{-1} should be dosed for ideal body weight (max bolus 500 mL)**

* lactate measurements are useful if available as they have prognostic ability if measured serially.

** Other bloods that may be indicated: coagulation studies, liver function tests, magnesium levels or any others indicated by the child's clinical picture.

*** Balanced (buffered) fluids are used in preference to 0.9% sodium chloride, but if not available, 0.9% sodium chloride should be used.

**** These are starting dose ranges for these inotropes, and increases may be necessary but should be guided by

PICU retrieval team/senior clinicians. Choice of inotropes is dictated by clinician preference, response to treatment and monitored parameters, and again decisions should be made in conjunction with PICU teams.

Useful links

The European Paediatric Advanced Life Support (EPALS) is an advanced course that trains healthcare professionals in the early recognition of the child in respiratory or circulatory failure and management of a cardiorespiratory arrest.

EPALS provides the knowledge and skills needed to prevent further deterioration and help to save young lives.

The EPALS course is a collaboration between Resuscitation Council UK and the European Resuscitation Council. It is approved by the Royal Colleges of Paediatric and Child Health (RCPCH), Emergency Medicine (RCEM), and Anaesthetics (RCoA), as well as the Association of Paediatric Anaesthetists (APAGBI).

Resuscitation Council UK Guidelines

Read all of the 2021 guidelines:
resus.org.uk/rcukgl21

Lifesaver and Lifesaver VR apps

Teach your friends and family lifesaving skills anytime, anywhere:
resus.org.uk/rcuklifesaver

iResus app

Get RCUK guidelines on the go:
resus.org.uk/rcukiresus

e-Lifesaver

Bring lifesaving training to your non-clinical staff:
resus.org.uk/rcukworkplace

Resuscitation Council UK courses

See all of the courses available:
resus.org.uk/rcukcourses

Follow us on Twitter

@ResusCouncilUK
twitter.com/ResusCouncilUK

RCUK membership

Get involved and join our community:
resus.org.uk/rcukmembers

Like us on Facebook

facebook.com/ResuscitationCouncilUK